The Kelalis-King-Belman Textbook of
Clinical Pediatric Urology
Study Guide

The Kelalis-King-Belman Textbook of
Clinical Pediatric Urology
Study Guide

Editor-in-Chief

Aseem R Shukla MD
Director of Pediatric Urology
Assistant Professor of Urologic Surgery and Pediatrics
University of Minnesota
Minneapolis, MN, USA

Associate Editors

Paul F Austin MD
Associate Professor of Surgery
St Louis Children's Hospital
Division of Urologic Surgery
Washington University School of Medicine
St Louis, MO, USA

CD Anthony Herndon MD
Associate Professor
Department of Surgery/Pediatrics
Division of Urology/Section Pediatric Urology
University of Alabama – Birmingham
Birmingham, AL, USA

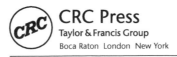

CRC Press
Taylor & Francis Group
Boca Raton London New York

CRC Press is an imprint of the
Taylor & Francis Group, an **informa** business

CRC Press
Taylor & Francis Group
6000 Broken Sound Parkway NW, Suite 300
Boca Raton, FL 33487-2742

First issued in paperback 2019

© 2009 by Taylor & Francis Group, LLC
CRC Press is an imprint of Taylor & Francis Group, an Informa business

No claim to original U.S. Government works

ISBN-13: 978-0-415-46016-3 (hbk)
ISBN-13: 978-0-367-38689-4 (pbk)

Visit the Taylor & Francis Web site at
http://www.taylorandfrancis.com

and the CRC Press Web site at
http://www.crcpress.com

Composition by Exeter Premedia Services Pvt Ltd, Chennai, India

Contents

Contributors

Mark C Adams MD FAAP
Professor of Urology and Pediatrics
Monroe Carell Jr Children's Hospital at Vanderbilt
Nashville, TN
USA

Kourosh Afshar MD FRCSC
Assistant Professor of Surgery (Urology)
University of British Columbia
Pediatric Urologist, BC Children's Hospital
Vancouver, BC
Canada

Jason W Anast MD
Resident in Urology
Department of Urology
Washington University School of Medicine
St Louis, MO
USA

Anthony Atala MD
The William Boyce Professor and Chair
Department of Urology
Wake Forest University School of Medicine
Winston-Salem, NC
USA

Paul F Austin MD FAAP
Associate Professor of Surgery
St Louis Children's Hospital
Division of Urologic Surgery
Washington University School of Medicine
St Louis, MO
USA

Linda A Baker MD
Associate Professor of Urology
Director of Pediatric Urology Unit
University of Texas Southwestern
Children's Medical Center at Dallas
Dallas, TX
USA

Stuart Bauer MD FAAP
Professor of Surgery
Director, Neuro-Urology
Surgery/Urology
Children's Hospital
Boston, MA
USA

John W Brock III MD
Director of Pediatric Urology
Vanderbilt University
Nashville, TN
USA

Mark P Cain MD FAAP
Associate Professor
James Whitcomb Riley Hospital for Children
Indiana University School of Medicine
Indianapolis, IN
USA

Anthony A Caldamone MD
Chief, Pediatric Urology
Hasbro Children's Hospital
Professor of Surgery, Urology
Brown University School of Medicine
Providence, RI
USA

Douglas A Canning MD
Director
Division of Pediatric Urology
Children's Hospital of Philadelphia
Philadelphia, PA
USA

Michael C Carr MD
Assistant Professor of Surgery and Urology
Division of Pediatric Urology
Children's Hospital of Pennsylvania
Philadelphia, PA
USA

Patrick Cartwright MD FAAP
Chief of Urology
Professor of Surgery and Pediatrics
University of Utah Health Sciences Center
Primary Children's Medical Center
Salt Lake City, UT
USA

Pasquale Casale MD
Division of Pediatric Urology
Children's Hospital of Pennsylvania
Philadelphia, PA
USA

Jorge R Caso MD
Resident in Urology
University of South Florida
Tampa, FL
USA

Marc Cendron MD
Associate Professor of Surgery (Urology)
Harvard School of Medicine
Department of Urology
Children's Hospital Boston
Boston, MA
USA

Earl Y Cheng MD
Associate Professor of Urology
Northwestern University's Feinberg
   School of Medicine
Department of Pediatric Urology
Children's Memorial Hospital
Chicago, IL
USA

Jeanne S Chow MD
Assistant Professor in Radiology
Harvard Medical School
Children's Hospital
Radiology
Boston, MA
USA

Douglass Clayton MD
Resident in Urology
University of Alabama – Birmingham
Birmingham, AL
USA

Christopher S Cooper MD
Associate Professor of Urology
Director
Pediatric Urology
University of Iowa and
Children's Hospital of Iowa
Iowa City, IA
USA

Lawrence Copelovitch MD
Division of Pediatric Nephrology
Children's Hospital of Philadelphia
Philadelphia, PA
USA

Douglas E Coplen MD
Director of Pediatric Urology
St Louis Children's Hospital
St Louis, MO
USA

William R DeFoor Jr MD
Assistant Professor
Division of Pediatric Urology
Cincinnati Children's Hospital Medical Center
Cincinnati, OH
USA

Romano T DeMarco MD FAAP
Pediatric Urology
Assistant Professor of Surgery
University of Missouri
Kansas City School of Medicine
Kansas City, MO
USA

Nafisa Dharamsi MD FRCSC
Pediatric Urology
Winnipeg Children's Hospital
Winnipeg, MB
Canada

David A Diamond MD
Associate Professor of Surgery
Harvard Medical School
Boston, MA
USA

Steven G Docimo MD
Professor and Director
Pediatric Urology
University of Pittsburgh School of Medicine
Children's Hospital of Pennsylvania
Pittsburgh, PA
USA

Jack S Elder MD
Chief, Department of Urology
Henry Ford Health System
Associate Director, Vattikuti Urology Institute
Children's Hospital of Michigan
Detroit, MI
USA

James M Elmore MD
Clinical Assistant Professor of Urology
Emory University School of Medicine
Atlanta, GA
USA

Walid Farhat MD
Assistant Professor
Department of Surgery
University of Toronto
Division of Urology
Hospital for Sick Children
Toronto, ON
Canada

Fernando Ferrer MD
Director
Pediatric Urologic Surgery
Surgeon-in-Chief
Connecticut Children's Medical Center
Hartford, CT
USA

T Ernesto Figueroa MD
Chief, Division of Pediatric Urology
New York Medical College
Valhalla, NY
USA

Israel Franco MD
Associate Professor of Urology
New York Medical College
Valhalla, NY
USA

Jens Goebel MD
Associate Professor of Pediatrics
Medical Director of Kidney Transplantation
Division of Nephrology and Hypertension
Cincinnati Children's Hospital Medical Center
Cincinnati, OH
USA

Richard W Grady MD
Associate Professor of Urology
Director
Clinical Research
University of Washington School of Medicine
Children's Hospital and Regional Medical Center
Seattle, WA
USA

Larry A Greenbaum MD PhD
Division Director
Pediatric Nephrology
Marcus Professor
Emory University and Children's Healthcare
  of Atlanta
Atlanta, GA
USA

Julie Franc-Guimond MD
Pediatric Urology
CHU Sainte-Justine
Montréal, PQ
Canada

CD Anthony Herndon MD FAAP FAS
Associate Professor
Department of Surgery/Pediatrics
Division of Urology/Section Pediatric Urology
University of Alabama – Birmingham
Birmingham, AL
USA

Anne-Marie Houle MD
CHU Sainte-Justine
Montréal, PQ
Canada

R Guy Hudson MD
Assistant Professor
Oregon Health and Science University
Pediatric Urology
Doembecher Children's Hospital
Portland, OR
USA

Douglas A Husmann MD
Chief and Professor of Urology
Mayo Clinic
Rochester, MN
USA

Douglas H Jamieson MBChB FRCPC
Clinical Assistant Professor of Radiology
British Columbia Children's Hospital
Vancouver, BC
Canada

Martin Kaefer MD
Associate Professor of Urology
Department of Pediatric Urology
Indiana University
Indianapolis, IN
USA

Bernard S Kaplan MD
Director of Pediatric Nephrology
Children's Hospital of Philadelphia
Philadelphia, PA
USA

George W Kaplan MD
Chief of Surgery
Children's Hospital and Health Center
San Diego, CA
USA

William E Kaplan MD
Head, Pediatric Urology
Associate Professor of Urology
Northwestern University's Feinberg School
  of Medicine
Division of Urology
Children's Memorial Hospital
Chicago, IL
USA

Michael A Keating MD
Medical Director
Spina Bifida Clinic
Department of Surgery
Division of Urology
Nemours Children's Clinic
Orlando, FL
USA

William A Kennedy II MD
Associate Professor
Department of Urology
Stanford University School of Medicine
Stanford, CA
USA

Antoine E Khoury MD
Professor of Urology
Chief, Division of Urology
Hospital for Sick Children
University of Toronto
Toronto, ON
Canada

Christina Kim MD
Assistant Professor of Surgery
Connecticut Children's Medical Center
Hartford, CT
USA

Andrew J Kirsch MD FAAP FACS
Professor of Urology
Emory University School of Medicine
Children's Healthcare of Atlanta
Atlanta, GA
USA

Thomas F Kolon MD FAAP
Assistant Professor of Urology
Children's Hospital of Philadelphia
Philadelphia, PA
USA

Martin A Koyle MD FAAP FACS
Chief, Division of Urology
Children's Hospital and Regional Medical Center
Seattle, WA
USA

Bradley P Kropp MD
Chief and Professor of Pediatric Urology
Department of Pediatric Urology
University of Oklahoma Health Sciences Center
Oklahoma City, OK
USA

Yegappan Lakshmanan MD FAAP
Assistant Professor, Pediatric Urology
Brady Urological Institute
Johns Hopkins Medical Institutions
Baltimore, MD
USA

Steven E Lerman MD
Assistant Professor of Urology
UCLA Urology
Los Angeles, CA
USA

Dennis B Liu MD
Assistant Professor of Urology
University of Toledo College of Medicine
Toledo, OH
USA

Armando J Lorenzo MD
Assistant Professor, Department of Surgery
(Urology)
Hospital for Sick Children
University of Toronto
Toronto, ON
Canada

Stephen Lukasewycz MD
Resident in Urology
Department of Urologic Surgery
University of Minnesota
Minneapolis, MN
USA

Irene M McAleer MD MBA FAAP FACS
Pediatric Urology
Children's Hospital Central California
Madeira, CA
USA

Gordon A McLorie MD
Chief, Pediatric Urology
Department of Urology
Wake Forest University School of Medicine
Winston-Salem, NC
USA

Andrew MacNeily MD FRSCS FAAP
Associate Professor of Surgery (Urology)
University of British Columbia
Vancouver, BC
Canada

Max Maizels MD
Director of Perinatal Urology
Feinberg School of Medicine at Northwestern
  University
Chicago, IL
USA

Scott R Manson PhD
Division of Urology
Washington University School of Medicine
St Louis, MO
USA

Sarah Marietti MD
Resident in Urology
University of Connecticut Affiliated Program in
  Urology
Hartford, CT
USA

Paul A Merguerian MD FRCSC FAAP
Professor of Surgery (Urology) and Pediatrics
Dartmouth-Hitchcock Medical Center
Dartmouth Medical School
Hanover, NH
USA

Kevin EC Meyers MD
Division of Pediatric Nephrology
Children's Hospital of Philadelphia
Philadelphia, PA
USA

Jennifer J Mickelson MD
Fellow in Pediatric Urology
Department of Pediatric Urology
Children's Memorial Hospital
Chicago, IL
USA

Eugene Minevich MD FAAP FACS
Associate Professor of Surgery
Cincinnati Children's Hospital Medical Center
Cincinnati, OH
USA

Rosalia Misseri MD
Assistant Professor of Pediatric Urology
Riley Children's Hospital
Indianapolis, IN
USA

Hiep T Nguyen MD
Co-Director
Center for Robotic Surgery
Director
Robotic Surgery Research and Training
Assistant Professor of Surgery (Urology)
Harvard Medical School
Boston, MA
USA

Michael Nguyen MD
Adjunct Clinical Instructor in Urology
Mayo Clinic College of Medicine
Pediatric Urology Associates
Phoenix, AZ
USA

Thomas E Novak MD
Fellow, Pediatric Urology
Brady Urological Institute
Johns Hopkins Medical Institutions
Baltimore, MD
USA

John M Park MD
Associate Professor, Urology
Director of Pediatric Urology
University of Michigan Medical School
Ann Arbor, MI
USA

João Luiz Pippi Salle MD PhD FAAP FRCSC
Professor, Division of Urology
Hospital for Sick Children
University of Toronto
Toronto, ON
Canada

Michael A Poch MD
Resident in Urology
The Warren Alpert Medical School of Brown
    University
Providence, RI
USA

Hans Pohl MD FAAP
Assistant Professor of Urology and Pediatrics
Department of Pediatric Urology
Children's National Medical Center
George Washington University School of
    Medicine
Washington, DC
USA

John C Pope IV MD
Associate Professor Urologic Surgery
Vanderbilt Children's Hospital
Nashville, TN
USA

Pramod P Reddy MD
Program Director
Pediatric Urology Fellowship
Division of Pediatric Urology
Cincinnati Children's Hospital Medical Center
Cincinnati, OH
USA

Richard C Rink MD FAAP
Chief Pediatric Urology
James Whitcomb Riley Hospital for Children
Indiana University School of Medicine
Indianapolis, IN
USA

Jonathan H Ross MD
Head of Section of Pediatric Urology
Glickman Urological Institute
Cleveland Clinic Childrens Hospital
Cleveland, OH
USA

H Gil Rushton MD FAAP
Chairman, Department of Pediatric Urology
Children's National Medical Center
Washington, DC
USA

Kara Sapperston MD
Resident in Urology
University of Utah College of Medicine
Salt Lake City, UT
USA

Ellen S Shapiro MD
Director Pediatric Urology
New York University School of Medicine
New York, NY
USA

Curtis A Sheldon MD
Professor of Surgery
Division of Pediatric Urology
Cincinnati Children's Hospital Medical Center
Cincinnati, OH
USA

Aseem R Shukla MD
Director of Pediatric Urology
Assistant Professor of Urologic Surgery
    and Pediatrics
University of Minnesota
Minneapolis, MN
USA

Steven J Skoog MD
Professor and Director
Pediatric Urology
Oregon Health and Science University
Doembecher Children's Hospital
Portland, OR
USA

Warren T Snodgrass MD FAAP
Professor of Urology
University of Southwestern Medical Center at
  Dallas
Dallas, TX
USA

Brent Snow MD FAAP
Professor of Surgery and Pediatrics
University of Utah Health Sciences Center
Primary Children's Medical Center
Salt Lake City, UT
USA

Howard M Snyder III MD
Associate Director
Pediatric Urology
Children's Hospital of Philadelphia
Philadelphia, PA
USA

John C Thomas MD
Adjunct Professor of Pharmacology
Vanderbilt University
Nashville, TN
USA

Julian Wan MD
Clinical Associate Professor of Urology
Pediatric Urology Division
University of Michigan Medical School
Ann Arbor, MI
USA

Elizabeth R Williams MD
Resident in Urology
Department of Urology
Washington University School of Medicine
St Louis, MO
USA

Ilene Wong MD
Resident
Department of Urology
Stanford University School of Medicine
Stanford, CA
USA

Hsi-Yang Wu MD
Assistant Professor of Urology
Children's Hospital of Pittsburgh
Pittsburgh, PA
USA

Richard N Yu MD PhD
Clinical Fellow in Urology
Children's Hospital
Boston, MA
USA

Stephen A Zderic MD
Professor of Surgery in Urology
University of Pennsylvania School of Medicine
Philadelphia, PA
USA

Preface

The *Kelalis-King-Belman Textbook of Clinical Pediatric Urology* is renowned as an invaluable, comprehensive resource for practicing pediatric urologists, fellows, and residents in training. The fifth edition of this classic textbook was published in 2007 and edited for the first time by Drs. Steven Docimo, Douglas Canning, and Antoine Khoury. This edition under new leadership continues to uphold the vaunted ideals of the previous textbook editions and firmly establishes itself as the definitive resource for the specialty.

Pediatric urology became the first subspecialty recognized by the American Board of Urology in the spring of 2008, as the first Certificate of Added Qualification was granted following a rigorous qualification process and written examination. That there is a paucity of sample questions and study guides available for the busy practitioner preparing for the certification exam, or for urology residents and medical students sitting for annual in-service exams, became apparent and prompted the publication of this text: *The Kelalis-King-Belman Textbook of Clinical Pediatric Urology Study Guide.*

This study guide is intended as a compendium to the authoritative textbook, and the entirety of the multiple choice questions presented herein are based on information relayed in the actual textbook. The embryology questions relevant to Chapters 19, 36, and 67 were included in Chapters 13–14 by the authors and are not separately listed here. No questions were submitted for Chapter 45, but relevant information is included in other related chapters.

Wherever possible, every effort was made to request the original authors of each chapter in the textbook to prepare questions that they felt encapsulated the key elements of their areas of expertise. The vast majority of the original authors participated in this exercise and we, the co-editors of this effort, are enormously grateful.

We express our admiration for the colossal endeavor of Steven Docimo, Douglas Canning, and Antoine Khoury to edit the textbook upon which we base our study guide. Our sincere appreciation, especially, to Steven Docimo for investing us with his confidence and guiding our efforts; and to Informa Healthcare for bringing forth what we hope will be a practical and valuable contribution to our discipline: pediatric urology

Aseem R Shukla
Paul F Austin
CD Anthony Herndon
July 2008

History and physical examination of the child

T Ernesto Figueroa and Aseem R Shukla

(Based on chapter written by T Ernesto Figueroa)

1. The most useful tool in the diagnosis of medical problems is:

   (a) Physical examination
   (b) Medical history
   (c) Reviews of system
   (d) Radiographic studies
   (e) Serum analysis

   Answer: (b) A properly obtained medical history accounts for 80% of the diagnostic process. The history taken initiates all further investigations and is critical to understanding and appreciating a medical condition.

2. Health Insurance Portability and Accountability Act (HIPAA) guidelines ensure that:

   (a) The patient receive comprehensive medical care despite the inability to pay for those services
   (b) Medical information regarding a pediatric patient be communicated to both the parents regardless of marital status or state of legal custody
   (c) Confidentiality and patient privacy are protected
   (d) Documentation in the medical record should indicate next of kin
   (e) Patients can designate power of attorney in case they are unable to make medical decisions for themselves

   Answer: (c) It is obligatory that the patient's confidentiality and privacy are protected, a federal oversight is established by the HIPAA guidelines. In the context of pediatric urology, this requires the physician to identify early on who will be the recipient of the medical information related to the child.

3. Common and effective distraction techniques include all of the following except:

   (a) The use of toys
   (b) Offering snacks
   (c) Talking to the child about their favorite activities
   (d) Timeout
   (e) Coloring books

   Answer: (d) The physician should be willing to listen and demonstrate empathy during a patient visit. If the child is disruptive and uncooperative, then distractive toys, coloring books or, at most, a gentle removal from the room may assist with history taking. Disciplining a child during a medical exam may set a negative precedent for future interactions.

4. The first sign of puberty in boys is usually:

   (a) The change of the voice
   (b) Axillary hair
   (c) The appearance of fine pubic hair
   (d) Growth of the penis and scrotum
   (e) Testicular growth

   Answer: (e) The first sign of puberty, usually around 11–12 years of age, is testicular growth.

Secondary sexual development, described by choices (a)–(d), follows after the onset of puberty. In females, the first sign of puberty is usually breast development, followed by the growth of pubic hair.

5. Menses usually occurs in which Tanner stage:

   (a) Stage 1
   (b) Stage 2
   (c) Stage 3
   (d) Stage 4
   (e) Stage 5

   Answer: (d) Menses heralds the onset of Tanner stage 4, and is associated with the development of coarse pubic hair and breast areola and papilla forming a secondary mound. Male children at Tanner stage 4 correspond to the same change in pubic hair, growth of axillary hair and voice changes.

6. Digital rectal examinations in children should routinely be performed in all of the following except:

   (a) A rectal exam should always be part of a complete physical examination

   (b) A 2-year-old child in acute urinary retention
   (c) A spinal cord injured patient
   (d) A chronically constipated child
   (e) A 12-year-old boy with spina bifida and urinary incontinence

   Answer: (a) The digital rectal examination is not routinely performed in children and is reserved for patients with pertinent complaints described in choices (b)–(e). This exam is performed using a well-lubricated, gloved fifth finger.

7. The greatest fear of a 5-year-old boy during examination is:

   (a) Separation from the parents
   (b) Loss of privacy
   (c) Undressing in front of strangers
   (d) Fear of needles
   (e) Bodily injury or castration

   Answer: (e) While separation anxiety predominates in children less than 3 years of age, fear of bodily injury or castration is most common in children between the ages of 4 and 6. Privacy becomes a preeminent issue in older children and adolescents.

Laboratory assessment of the pediatric urologic patient

2

Paul F Austin

(Based on chapter written by Paul F Austin and Erica J Traxel)

1. A 6-year-old girl is referred to you by her pediatrician for microscopic hematuria found on urine dipstick during a work-up for an upper respiratory infection. Your next step is to:

    (a) Obtain a renal and bladder ultrasound
    (b) Perform cystoscopy
    (c) Obtain a microscopic urinalysis
    (d) Obtain a urine culture
    (e) Obtain a serum basic metabolic panel

    Answer: (c) Urine dipstick results will often have false-positive results. Although the other tests may be necessary depending on the history and further work-up, a microscopic urinalysis will verify that red blood cells (RBCs) are indeed present.

2. With the presence of dysmorphic RBCs on microscopic urinalysis, the next step would be:

    (a) Obtain a renal and bladder ultrasound
    (b) Perform cystoscopy
    (c) Repeat the microscopic urinalysis in 1 week
    (d) Obtain a urine culture
    (e) Obtain a complete blood count (CBC), basic metabolic panel, C3 level, antistreptolysin-O (ASO) titer and antinuclear antibody test (ANA)

    Answer: (e) Microscopic abnormal shaped RBCs or dysmorphic RBCs are more commonly associated with nephrologic causes of hematuria, and normal shaped or eumorphic RBCs are more commonly associated with urologic causes. This panel of serum tests is selectively performed if renal and bladder sonography are negative and the urine microscopy suggests a nephrologic origin. These may subsequently indicate hematologic- or immunologic-mediated diseases affecting the kidney.

3. An asymptomatic newborn is noted to have an enlarged left hemi-scrotum with a transilluminable, nonreducible mass. A serum alpha-fetoprotein (AFP) level was drawn and measured 48,000 ng/ml. Your next step is:

    (a) Reassurance and observation
    (b) Scrotal exploration with possible left radical orchiectomy
    (c) CT scan
    (d) CBC, beta human chorionic gonadotropin (HCG), lactate dehydrogenase (LDH) and placental alkaline phosphatase (PLAP)
    (e) Scrotal U/S

    Answer: (a) AFP at birth is relatively high and will remain so for the first several months of life, due to the yolk sac elements present during gestation. In this example, the newborn has a neonatal hydrocele and family reassurance, and observation of the neonatal hydrocele is all that is necessary.

4. A 14-year-old boy presents for follow-up after an extracorporeal shock wave lithotripsy

(ESWL) for an 8 mm right renal calculus. The patient is "stone free" on kidneys, ureter, bladder X-ray (KUB) and sonographic imaging. The next step is:

(a) Reassurance and observation
(b) Metabolic evaluation
(c) CT scan
(d) Spot urine calcium/creatinine ratio
(e) Initiate high-fluid therapy

Answer: (b) The prevalence of nephrolithiasis in children is less than in the adult population and extensive laboratory assessment is recommended upon initial presentation. As opposed to the adult patient, nephrolithiasis in the pediatric population is more likely attributable to a metabolic abnormality. Standard metabolic evaluation for pediatric nephrolithiasis includes serum tests and a 24-hour urine study. A serum CBC, electrolytes, bicarbonate, calcium, phosphorus, blood urea nitrogen (BUN), creatinine, alkaline phosphatase, magnesium, and uric acid should be obtained. A 24-hour urine collection should be obtained on a regular diet to check calcium, phosphorus, magnesium, oxalate, sodium, uric acid, citrate, cystine, creatinine, and volume.

5. You are called to the nursery for consultation regarding a newborn with ambiguous genitalia. Inspection and examination of the genitalia reveals a phallic structure with a severe hypospadias and impalpable gonads. The most critical test in the work-up is:

(a) Karyotype
(b) Electrolytes
(c) Genitogram

(d) 17-OH progesterone
(e) Müllerian inhibiting substance (MIS)

Answer: (d) The most common intersex condition is congenital adrenal hyperplasia (CAH). It is important to identify CAH early to prevent any electrolyte and metabolic imbalances such as "salt-wasting". Although the other tests are important in the work-up of a child with intersex, serum 17-OH progesterone is critical because elevated levels identify CAH and would direct prompt intervention.

6. An 18-month-old male is referred for bilateral, nonpalpable cryptorchidism. Appropriate laboratory testing would include consideration of which of the following:

(a) Karyotype
(b) Serum testosterone and gonadotropins
(c) HCG stimulation test
(d) MIS
(e) All of the above

Answer: (e) A karyotype should be performed to rule out an intersex condition. Serum testosterone levels may be obtained but would be low at this age and must be referenced to the levels of the gonadotropins to have any relevance. (Remember there is normal elevation of serum testosterone at 2–3 months of age as well as at puberty.) An HCG stimulation test is a good way of checking for testosterone production from any testicular tissue. Finally, measuring serum MIS levels that are produced by the Sertoli cell is the most sensitive indicator of testicular presence. Unfortunately, the MIS enzyme-linked immunosorbent assay (ELISA) is not readily available in most labs.

Fetal urology and prenatal diagnosis

3

CD Anthony Herndon

(Based on chapter written by Dave Thomas)

1. During the third trimester, urine constitutes what percentage of amniotic fluid?

   (a) 50%
   (b) 100%
   (c) 70%
   (d) 90%
   (e) 10%

   Answer: (d)   By the third trimester, urine production equals 30–40 ml/h and comprises up to 90% of amniotic fluid volume. (Page 19)

2. Amniotic fluid is vital for fetal lung development secondary to:

   (a) Does not play a role
   (b) Mechanical properties of stenting open airways
   (c) Provides a liquid surface that decreases surface tension
   (d) Provides potential growth factors for aveoli

   Answer: (b) and (d)   Amniotic fluid provides growth factors for fetal lung development in addition to the mechanical properties of stenting open the airways. (Page 20)

3. Following birth, an increase in renal perfusion occurs which results in estimated glomerular filtration rate (GFR) to be:

   (a) $75\,ml/1.73\,m^2$
   (b) $100\,ml/1.73\,m^2$
   (c) $30\,ml/1.73\,m^2$
   (d) $125\,ml/1.73\,m^2$
   (e) $5\,ml/1.73\,m^2$

   Answer: (c)   Despite a dramatic increase in renal perfusion pressure, the initial GFR is quite low at $30\,ml/m^2$. At two years of life it approaches $125\,ml/m^2$. (Page 20)

4. In patients with suspected bladder outlet obstruction, a poor prognosis may be predicted for the following:

   (a) Bladder distention identified <24 weeks
   (b) Thickened bladder wall
   (c) Anteroposterior (AP) diameter renal pelvis diameter >10 mm
   (d) Male fetus
   (e) All of the above

   Answer: (e)   All of the above, plus oligohydramnios are believed to be a bad prognostic indicator for early-onset renal deterioration. (Page 22)

5. Prenatal ultrasound findings which may be consistent with lower urinary tract pathology include:

   (a) Ureterocele
   (b) Visualization of a ureter
   (c) Thickened bladder wall
   (d) Multicystic dysplastic kidney (MCDK)
   (e) All of the above

   Answer: (e)   All of the above including MCDK may be associated with pathology at the bladder level. Vesicoureteral reflux (VUR) is associated with MCDK in up to 40% of patients. (Page 26)

6. Vesicoureteral reflux that is detected in patients with prenatal hydronephrosis:

   (a) Usually occurs in boys
   (b) Usually occurs in girls
   (c) Tends to be low grade and unilateral
   (d) Tends to be high grade and bilateral
   (e) Demonstrates a high spontaneous resolution rate

Answer: (a) and (e) Vesicoureteral reflux that is detected prenatally with hydronephrosis is more common in boys, tends to be high grade and bilateral, and resolves spontaneously at a rate higher than expected. Girls tend to present with urinary tract infections postnatally and the majority of their reflux is low grade.

In-office ultrasonography

Dennis Liu and Max Maizels

4

1. Which of the following ultrasound probes would be most appropriate to image the kidney of a large 14-year-old boy?

   (a) 3 mHz
   (b) 5 mHz
   (c) 7.5 mHz
   (d) 10 mHz
   (e) Any of the above probes would be appropriate

   Answer: (a)   The lower the mHz of the probe, the better tissue penetrance is obtained. In order to image the kidneys in a large 14-year-old child, the 3 Mhz probe offers the best tissue penetrance and would be the best choice. (Page 35)

2. An 18-month-old child is seen in the office for an in-office ultrasound (IOUS). During the exam, an overlying rib obscures the child's left kidney and she becomes increasingly agitated and uncooperative. Which of the following positions is optimal to obtain an image of this kidney?

   (a) Supine with the probe placed in laterally along the axillary line
   (b) Left lateral decubitus position
   (c) Prone position
   (d) Have the caregiver hold the child and image the kidney from the prone position
   (e) Supine with the probe anteriorly in an intercostal space

   Answer: (d)   The prone position is the best position to image a kidney obscured by ribs.

In an uncooperative younger child, the comfort of being held by the caregiver will often calm the child down and allow a better exam. (Page 36)

3. A 7-year-old girl is referred to the office for unilateral Grade 1 hydronephrosis. An IOUS is performed which confirms the finding of right hydronephrosis. All of the following manuevers on IOUS would help make the diagnosis of vesicoureteral reflux (VUR) except for:

   (a) Imaging of the bladder transversely while full
   (b) Imaging of the bladder transversely after voiding
   (c) Imaging of the bladder parasagittally from the right
   (d) Imaging of the bladder parasagittally from the left
   (e) Imaging of the kidneys after voiding

   Answer: (c)   Use of IOUS is helpful in certain situations to delineate unilateral hydronephrosis due to VUR from ureteropelvic junction obstruction. Resolution of hydronephrosis after voiding would favor a diagnosis of VUR while persistence of unilateral hydronephrosis after voiding would suggest possible ureteropelvic junction (UPJ) obstruction. (Page 38) Likewise, imaging for dilated distal ureters with a full bladder and resolution after voiding would also be suggestive of VUR. This is best done either transversely (ureters located posterior to the bladder) or viewed longitudinally by viewing the ureter from the contralateral parasagittal view of the bladder. Thus, left parasagittal views of the bladder would be used to image the right ureter. (Page 36)

4. A two-month-old child is seen in the office for evaluation of severe unilateral hydronephrosis. You perform an IOUS. Which of the following findings would be suggestive of a severely obstructed UPJ rather than a multicystic dysplastic kidney?

   (a) An echogenic contralateral kidney
   (b) Contiguity of the dilated renal pelvis and dilated calyces
   (c) Involution of the kidney on serial follow-up exams
   (d) Elongated kidney without reniform shape with multiple cysts
   (e) All of the above

   Answer: (b) The differentiation between a severely obstructed kidney and a multicystic dysplastic kidney (MCDK) can be challenging. The key differential feature is the contiguity of the dilated renal pelvis with the dilated calyces that is not seen in a MCDK and the lack of involution of the severely obstructed kidney on serial exams. Furthermore, additional features suggestive of a MCDK include: an echogenic elongated kidney without reniform shape; multiple noncommunicating cysts; a contralateral echogenic kidney; and perhaps most importantly, involution of the MCDK over time. (Page 40)

5. An IOUS is performed on routine follow-up on a 14-day-old neonate found to have bilateral prenatal sonographically evident renal pelvis (SERP). Examination of the bladder ultrasound demonstrates echogenic material within the bladder lumen. Which of the following is most likely responsible for this finding?

   (a) Bladder calculi
   (b) Phosphate crystals

   (c) Uric acid crystals
   (d) Tamm-Horsfall protein
   (e) Hypercalcuria

   Answer: (d) The echogenic characteristic of a neonate's bladder is usually due to the Tamm-Horsfall protein. The normal urine in older children is echolucent.

6. A 6-year-old girl is seen in the office for evaluation of incontinence and recurrent urinary tract infections (UTIs). An IOUS is performed and her bladder capacity is calculated. What is the expected bladder capacity of a 6-year-old child?

   (a) 140 ml
   (b) 180 ml
   (c) 240 ml
   (d) 280 ml
   (e) 340 ml

   Answer: (c) The formula to estimate the bladder capacity is as follows: Bladder capacity (ounces) = age (years) + 2. To convert ounces to ml, one multiples the capacity by 30. Thus, a 6-year-old child should have a bladder capacity of 240 ml (or 8 ounces). (Page 48)

7. The following ultrasound is obtained on a 2-week-old neonate as follow-up for prenatally detected right SERP. Which of the following is the likely diagnosis?

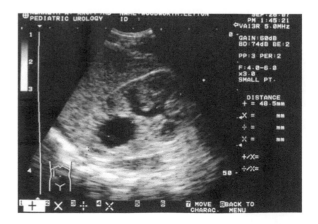

(a) Normal right kidney without hydro-nephrosis

(b) Right kidney with Society of Fetal Urology (SFU) Grade 2 hydronephrosis

(c) Right kidney SFU Grade 4 hydro-nephrosis

(d) Right kidney with duplex system and hydronephrosis of upper pole moiety

(e) Right kidney with duplex system and hydronephrosis of lower pole moiety

Answer: (d)   This ultrasound image obtained in the office represents an ideal way to follow-up on prenatally detected SERP. This kidney likely has a duplex system as evidenced by separation of the central echogenic complex (CEC). The upper pole in a duplex system is seen laterally on a sagittal view of the kidney and the lower pole medially. In this case, hydronephrosis is seen in the upper pole moiety. (Pages 37, 40, 44)

8. An IOUS is obtained in the office on a 1-month-old child as follow-up for prenatally detected SERP. The following ultrasound is obtained. What best describes the ultrsound finding?

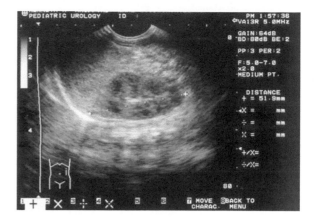

(a) Normal kidney

(b) SFU Grade 1 hydronephrosis

(c) SFU Grade 2 hydronephrosis

(d) SFU Grade 3 hydronephrosis

(e) SFU Grade 4 hydronephrosis

Answer: (a)   This is an image of a normal right kidney. The hypoechoic pockets seen between the renal cortex and renal sinus are prominent renal pyramids typically seen in children. These are not to be confused with hydronephrosis as there appears to be no connection with the renal pelvis. Furthermore, there is no evidence of dilation within the CEC. (Page 37)

Pediatric renal nuclear medicine 5

Aseem R Shukla

(Based on chapter written by Martin Charron)

1. The radioactive tracer providing the most effective relative measure of glomerular filtration rate (GFR) in children more than 5 year of age is:

   (a) ^{99m}Tc-diethylenetriaminepentaacetic acid (DTPA)
   (b) ^{99m}Tc-mercaptoacetyl triglycine (MAG3)
   (c) ^{131}I- or ^{123}I-orthoiodohippurate (OIH)
   (d) ^{99m}Tc-dimercaptosuccinic acid (DMSA)
   (e) ^{131}I radioiodine

   Answer: (a) ^{99m}Tc DTPA has >95% excretion by glomerular filtration and becomes a reliable method of measuring relative function on each side and measuring GFR in children more than 5 years of age. DTPA is taken up by the kidney through glomerular filtration and is not secreted or reabsorbed by the renal tubules. Once it reaches the kidney, about 20% is accumulated and the remainder flows away.

2. All of the following regarding ^{99m}Tc MAG3 are true except:

   (a) It is taken up in the proximal tubules
   (b) It shows high plasma protein binding and readily filters through the glomerular membrane
   (c) A high extraction fraction makes high-resolution imaging possible
   (d) Differential renal function analysis may be difficult if one kidney has markedly decreased or delayed renal function
   (e) A poorly functioning renal unit renders a MAG3 study unreliable due to a poor response to furosemide administered during the exam

   Answer: (b) MAG3 does bind with plasma protein, but does not filter through the glomerular membrane, giving it a high extraction fraction and resolution. MAG3 is the radiotracer of choice for its reliable estimation of differential renal function and renal clearance. The remainder of the choices are all true.

3. The ^{99m}Tc DMSA is ideal for the evaluation of acute pyelonephritis because:

   (a) It accumulates in the proximal renal tubules
   (b) Impaired renal cortex and space-occupying lesions are depicted as hyperactive areas with DMSA
   (c) DMSA accurately differentiates between a renal scar or acute pyelonephritic changes
   (d) The DMSA scan detects pyelonephritic changes while determining the presence of a ureteropelvic junction obstruction
   (e) Acute pyelonephritis appears as a nonsegmental reduction in cortical accumulation of DMSA

   Answer: (e) DMSA accumulates in functioning renal cortical tissue for a prolonged period and impaired areas appear hypoactive. The DMSA scan is a preferred adjunct in the diagnosis of a child with pyelonephritis, but does not provide reliable assessment of urinary obstruction. While hypoactive areas may reflect acute pyelonephritis, follow-up imaging is necessary to determine if a previously detected lesion is a permanent parenchymal abnormality, such as a renal scar.

Prenatal and postnatal urologic emergencies

6

Sarah Marietti and Fernando Ferrer
(Based on chapter written by Patrick McKenna and Fernando Ferrer)

1. All of the following are findings of bladder exstrophy by screening ultrasound except:

   (a) Lower abdominal bulge
   (b) Low set umbilicus
   (c) Nonvisualization of the bladder
   (d) Hydronephrosis
   (e) Small penis

   Answer: (d) Studies have identified five common prenatal finding on ultrasound to suggest bladder exstrophy: inability to visualize bladder on multiple ultrasounds, lower abdominal bulge, small penis with anteriorly placed scrotum, low set umbilicus, and abnormal widening of the iliac crests. Although hydronephrosis can be found in addition to bladder exstrophy, it is not indicative of the diagnosis.

2. In regards to ambiguous genitalia which of the following is true?

   (a) The most common cause is mixed gonadal dysgenesis
   (b) The most common enzyme deficiency in congenital adrenal hyperplasia (CAH) is 11B-hydroxylase
   (c) CAH may be life-threatening secondary to low serum potassium and high serum sodium levels
   (d) 17-hydroxyprogesterone levels will be elevated when CAH is present

   (e) CAH is the most likely diagnosis when the karyotype is 46XX and uterus is not visualized on ultrasound

   Answer: (d) The most common cause of ambiguous genitalia is CAH. The most common enzyme deficiency associated with CAH is 21-hydoxylase deficiency. The second most common deficiency is 11-hydroxylase. Lastly, 3beta-hydroxysteroid dehydrogenase can also cause CAH but is extremely rare. CAH, if unrecognized and untreated, is life threatening in the salt-waster secondary to poor feeding, dehydration, and hyperkalemia leading to arrhythmias and shock. When the cause is 21-hydroxylase, blood tests for 17-hydroxyprogesterone and progesterone will be elevated. These tests should be ordered after day 2 of life because they may be falsely elevated early in life from the stress of delivery. 45XX CAH patients will still have Müllerian ducal structures, such as a uterus, visible on pelvic ultrasound.

3. In regards to neonatal circumcision:

   (a) Amputation is usually associated with plastibell clamp use
   (b) The removed penile skin should be used to repair a degloving injury
   (c) If urethral injury occurs, a catheter should be placed to allow healing by secondary intention

(d) Bleeding should be cauterized while the metallic clamp is in place

Answer: (b) The mogan clamp is more commonly associated with amputation of the glans as the clamp may be placed at an angle drawing the frenulum and the glans up into the clamp. The removed penile skin, if preserved, may be used to repair an injury. Injuries involving the urethra should be managed by immediate reconstruction within hours of the injury. Repairs performed days after the injury have been reported but with decreased success rates. If bleeding is cauterized while the metallic clamp is in place, the current may be transferred to the clamp causing unintentional penile cauterization.

4. Multicystic dysplastic kidney (MCDK):

   (a) Is associated with contralateral renal anomaly in 50% of patients
   (b) Is diagnosed by ultrasound revealing multiple connected cysts
   (c) Is typically followed with serial ultrasounds for spontaneous regression
   (d) When associated with vesicoureteral reflux is usually grade IV–V

Answer: (c) MCDK is usually unilateral and associated with contralateral anomalies 25% of the time. The contralateral kidney anomaly is most commonly UPJ obstruction or vesicoureteral reflux. When reflux is present (25% of the time), the majority are low grade and most will resolve spontaneously. Ultrasound should demonstrate nonconnected cysts and should be done serially to verify regression. In the past, nephrectomy was the recommended treatment based on reports of malignancy within these kidneys. However, chance of malignancy is extremely low, making conservative management standard.

5. The most common solid malignancy in the neonate is:

   (a) Neuroblastoma

(b) Wilms' tumor
(c) Renal cell carcinoma
(d) Congenital mesoblastic nephroma

Answer: (d) Neuroblastoma is the most common solid malignancy in the neonate. Wilms' tumors are the most common renal tumors in children but rarely occur in the neonate. Renal cell carcinoma is rare in young children. However, in children older than 10 years of age, presenting with a solid renal mass, 50% will be of renal cell origin. Congenital mesoblastic nephroma is the most common solid renal mass in the neonate. Many are detected prenatally or in the first month after birth. The cellular variant is capable of metastasis and once this occurs the child will require chemotherapy. The classic variant is not capable of metastasis and nephrectomy alone is the treatment of choice.

6. When treating a presumptive patient with CAH with prenatal corticosteroids, what fraction of patients are not expected to benefit?

   (a) $1/4$
   (b) $1/2$
   (c) $1/8$
   (d) $7/8$
   (e) $3/4$

Answer: (d) CAH is inherited in an autosomal recessive fashion which gives a 25% likelihood of being afflicted with the disease. Corticosteroids are given early in the first trimester in an attempt to prevent virilization of the external genitalia. In that 50% of fetuses will be male, $7/8$ of recipients will not benefit from treatment.

7. Anorectal malformations are associated with a urologic abnormality in 20–60% of patients. One of these, neuropathic bladder, should be studied early in the evaluation process with urodynamics. What is the expected etiology of a neuropathic bladder in this population?

   (a) Tethered cord

(b) Spina bifida
(c) Lipomeningocele
(d) Syrinx
(e) Myelomeningocele

Answer: (a) When vertebral anomalies are present, a tethered spinal cord is the most common etiology of a neuropathic bladder in this population. Although the other processes may occur, it is not an anticipated finding in this population.

8. In the newborn nursery on routine examination 5 hours after a prolonged vaginal delivery, an erythematous, firm and tender right hemiscrotum is discovered. On reviewing the delivery examination notes, both testes were thought to be present at birth and the scrotum was normal. The next step should be:

(a) Allow discharge home
(b) Observation in the nursery for 24 hours
(c) Immediate exploration for suspected testicular torsion
(d) Attempt to detorse at the bedside and then obtain an ultrasound
(e) Obtain a KUB radiograph

Answer: (c) Neonatal torsion may present in the early postdelivery time period. It is hallmarked by a change in the scrotal exam as compared to immediate delivery. In this setting, i.e. <6 hours, immediate exploration is warranted. The pathogenesis is likely to be extravaginal torsion. Bilateral inguinal incisions are most commonly used because of the increased incidence of a patent process. Also, in rare cases, a testicular tumor is responsible for the torsion of the testicle.

9. When evaluating a newborn with ambiguous genitalia, the phallic structure is a Prader III with a perineal hypospadias. Labioscrotal folds are fused. Neither gonad is palpable.

Which of the following should be performed immediately:

(a) Ultrasound of pelvis
(b) Sequential multi-channel analysis (SMA)-7
(c) Karyotype
(d) Genitogram
(e) 17-hydroxyprogesterone level

Answer: (b) Although imperative for the correct diagnosis, the karyotype, steroid pathway precursor studies and radiologic imaging do not need to be performed immediately. Salt wasting CAH can be fatal if not detected in the newborn time period.

10. During the evaluation of gross hematuria for a 1-week-old premature infant born to a diabetic mother, a renal ultrasound reveals an edematous kidney with minimal but present arterial wave form. A renal scan reveals an enlarged kidney with decreased blood flow and function. The most likely diagnosis is:

(a) Adrenal hemorrhage
(b) Renal artery thrombosis
(c) Renal trauma secondary to prolonged vaginal delivery
(d) Congenital mesoblastic nephroma
(e) Renal vein thrombosis

Answer: (e) Although all of these may result in gross hematuria in the neonate, given the above history, renal vein thrombosis is the most likely etiology. Infants of diabetic mothers may be initially dehydrated and result in renal vein thrombosis. A renal ultrasound of renal artery thrombosis typically does not demonstrate an edematous kidney and the renal scan will reveal no function and no blood flow. The management of renal vein thrombosis may consist of hydration and/ or anticoagulants depending on the clinical situation.

Urinary tract infections in children

Hans Pohl and H Gil Rushton

1. All of the following are true of bacteriuria except:

(a) Declines with increasing age
   (b) More common in boys aged >10 years than in girls aged >10 years
   (c) Male to female predominance (2.5:1) in first year of life
   (d) Treatment with short-term oral antibiotics does not usually provide lasting resolution of occult bacteriuria
   (e) Ten times more common in uncircumcised than in circumcised boys

Answer: (b) The results of several large epidemiological studies have shown that bacteriuria occurs in 1–1.4% of neonates, most of those being uncircumcised boys under 6 months of age. The male:female ratio is reversed in older children. In a prospective screening study in Sweden of 3581 infants who underwent suprapubic aspiration, the incidence of occult bacteriuria was 2.5% in boys and 0.9% in girls. Symptomatic urinary tract infection (UTI) occurred with equal frequency (1.2% of boys and 1.1% of girls) in both sexes. The male predominance declines after the first year of life, such that later in childhood, bacteriuria, whether occult or symptomatic, is very unlikely in boys as compared with girls.

2. All of the following are true of UTIs except:

(a) Risk of recurrent UTI is approximately 25% in infants
   (b) Risk of recurrent UTIs in older girls approaches 60%
   (c) Girls with a history of bacilluria have a greater incidence of bacilluria of pregnancy than healthy controls
   (d) Children born to bacilluric women do not have a greater risk of bacilluria themselves
   (e) Up to two-thirds of boys with symptomatic UTIs will present with temperature >38°C

Answer: (d) Prospective studies have shown that some children carry a lifelong propensity towards UTI. One study found a greater incidence of bacteriuria during pregnancy among girls with a childhood history of bacteriuria as compared to healthy controls (64% and 27%, respectively). This propensity persisted in the children born to bacteriuric women, whereas none of the children born to healthy controls demonstrated bacteriuria.

3. Which of the following is true:

(a) An uncircumcised adolescent boy is more likely to acquire a UTI with *Proteus* than with *E. coli*
   (b) Neonatal boys are at similar risk for UTI caused by *E. coli* when compared with neonatal girls
   (c) Adolescent girls are at greatest risk of streptococcal UTIs
   (d) *Klebsiella* is a frequent cause of UTI in older children

(e) Struvite stones are associated with *Pseudomonas* UTIs

Answer: (a) Although the majority of UTIs are caused by *E. coli*, the bacteriologic findings in the Goteborg bacteriuria study suggest that the environmental factors which determine what type of bacteria cause UTIs are in turn influenced by age and gender.

4. Choose the best response regarding the importance of bacterial virulence factors:

   (a) K capsular antigens, hemolysin and aerobactin are critical for tissue invasion by bacteria
   (b) Only mannose-resistant fimbria are important in cell surface attachment
   (c) The presence of *P. fimbria* predisposes to nonreflux pyelonephritis
   (d) Hemolysin-producing *E. coli* are more virulent due to their ability to resist phagocytosis
   (e) Lewis blood group secretors are more likely to be infected by P. fimbriated strains of *E. coli*

Answer: (c) *P. fimbria* poses specific adhesion molecules that are most associated with nonreflux pyelonephritis. Epidemiological studies in children have provided considerable evidence that the presence of *P. fimbriae* on *E. coli* is a significant virulence factor, particularly in upper UTIs. These studies have shown that 76–94% of pyelonephritogenic strains of *E. coli* are P. fimbriated compared with 19–23% of cystitis strains, 14–18% of strains isolated from patients with asymptomatic bacteriuria, and 7–16% of fecal isolate strains.

5. Regarding the role of *P. fimbria* in the etiology of UTIs choose the true answer:

   (a) *P. fimbria* predispose to febrile UTIs only by promoting bacterial tropism (attachment) to renal parenchyma

   (b) P. fimbrial receptors are "not exposed" and are located within the connective tissue that supports the uroepithelium
   (c) Some soluble urinary proteins may actually promote bacterial adherence by binding to *P. fimbria*
   (d) A bacterium's phenotype is invariable, thus it reliably predicts the organism's ability to colonize the upper urinary tract
   (e) *P. fimbria* may be differentiated by different tip antigens which impart selectivity for uroepithelial cells in different locations of the urinary tract

Answer: (e) Further research has identified that not all *P. fimbria* are alike. Proteins located at the tip (G-tip proteins, or tip adhesins) determine the fimbria's specific attachment properties. Three classes have been identified, of which only class II and class III *P. fimbria* have uropathogenic potential. In vitro studies have found that the class III *P. fimbria* bind receptors found in higher density on bladder uroepithelium. In contrast, class II tip adhesins may be more important in the evolution of acute pyelonephritis by virtue of an increased density of class II specific receptors located on the uroepithelium of the upper urinary tract.

6. All of the following are host risk factors for the development of UTI except one:

   (a) Perineal or perimeatal colonization
   (b) Presence of low-grade vesicoureteral reflux (VUR)
   (c) Presence of P. fimbriated *E. coli* in fecal isolates
   (d) Absence of secreted antigens which assist in clearing bacteria from the urinary tract
   (e) Delayed micturition and constipation

Answer: (b) VUR in and of itself does not increase a child's risk for UTI, instead should UTI occur, the presence of VUR – particularly of higher grades – can increase the risk for acquired renal cortical abnormalities.

7. A 7-year-old Hispanic girl recently immigrated to the United States presents with frequent urination (sometimes hourly). Her mother specifically denies posturing maneuvers. She has no daytime incontinence and no history of fecal soiling. She remains dry throughout the night. Her physical exam and urinalysis are both normal. Choose the best diagnosis:

  (a) Lazy bladder syndrome
  (b) Occult spina bifida
  (c) Bacterial cystitis
  (d) Daytime frequency syndrome
  (e) Urgency-frequency syndrome

Answer: (d)   The key feature of this child's voiding complaints is the high frequency with which she is voiding throughout the day, without other features of dysfunctional elimination such as posturing, wetting or constipation and fecal soiling. The daytime frequency syndrome is selflimiting and not associated with an increased risk for UTI.

8. An 8-year-old girl presents for evaluation of culture documented recurrent UTIs characterized by dysuria and wetting in the absence of fevers. Her parents note that she often crosses her legs and urgently seeks the toilet. She has infrequent bowel movements and has recently had one or two episodes of fecal soiling. Her physical exam and urinalysis are both normal. Choose the best diagnosis:

  (a) Dysfunctional/infrequent voider
  (b) Detrusor hyperreflexia with urge incontinence
  (c) Normal for her age
  (d) Daytime frequency syndrome
  (e) Ectopic ureter

Answer: (a)   This child suffers from urgency and urge incontinence, but the coexistence of constipation suggests that she has a more pervasive elimination problem than simple bladder overactivity.

9. All of the following regarding elimination and the risk of UTIs are true except:

  (a) Greater than 50% of children being evaluated for UTI will demonstrate squatting, delayed micturition and/or constipation
  (b) A majority of girls with occult bacilluria have urodynamic evidence of dysfunctional bladders
  (c) Dysfunctional voiding rarely contributes to the risk of UTI in children with anatomically normal urinary tracts
  (d) Placing a child with a history of UTI on oral fiber supplements significantly reduces the likelihood of further infections
  (e) Children with dysfunctional voiding often have urinary leakage despite large bladder capacities

Answer: (c)   The presence of dysfunctional elimination should be considered, evaluated for and treated in any child presenting with UTI and/or VUR, particularly since it has been determined by a number of studies that both the risk of recurrent UTI and VUR resolution are beneficially influenced by treating abnormal elimination.

10. Choose the best response regarding reflux nephropathy:

  (a) Experimental models have confirmed the detrimental effect of sterile primary urinary reflux on renal parenchyma
  (b) Focal acquired renal scarring is most likely to occur at polar regions in association with compound calyces
  (c) Among children with dimercaptosuccinic acid (DMSA) scan documented acute pyelonephritis, those with VUR are more likely to develop newly acquired renal scarring than those without
  (d) In kidneys with severe VUR, clinical studies have demonstrated progressive acquired renal scarring despite successful control of urinary infection with antibiotic prophylaxis

(e) Renal papilla are inherently susceptible to invasion by pyelonephritogenic *E. coli*

Answer: (e)   Primary, sterile reflux of urine does not harm the renal parenchyma and is the basis for placing children on antibiotic prophylaxis while awaiting resolution of VUR. Acquired renal cortical abnormalities more commonly occur on the upper and lower poles of the kidney, as a consequence of differences in papillary configuration which permits influx of urine into the parenchyma. The risk of renal scarring (approx 40%) is no different among children with acute pyelonephritis (APN) who have VUR as compared with those who do not have VUR.

11. Choose the false statement regarding post-pyelonephritic renal scarring:

   (a) Hypertension is most common in children with bilateral acquired renal scars
   (b) All renal scarring associated with severe reflux is acquired
   (c) The incidence of hypertension in children with acquired renal scarring increases with age
   (d) Not all patients with acquired renal scarring suffer hypertension
   (e) Prenatally detected reflux may be associated with significant functional abnormalities even in the absence of infection

Answer: (b)   When performed prior to the first febrile UTI, DMSA renal scans have shown renal cortical abnormalities – particularly in kidneys associated with high grades of VUR – which can only be ascribed to defects during induction of renal tissue.

12. Which child does not require radiographic evaluation following a UTI:

   (a) A 2-year-old uncircumcised boy with a positive screening urine culture confirmed by cathed specimen

   (b) A 2-year-old girl with high fevers and a positive culture obtained by catheterization
   (c) A 5-year-old girl with a nonfebrile urine culture documented UTI and a history of fecal soiling and enuresis
   (d) A 7-year-old girl with three nonfebrile culture documented UTIs over the last 2 years and a normal voiding history
   (e) A 7-year-old boy with his first culture documented UTI and a normal voiding history

Answer: (d)   Children with UTI are evaluated in order to identify urological abnormalities that place that child at risk for progressive renal dysfunction should recurrent infection occur. In the case of scenario (d), the child has demonstrated no propensity for acquired renal cortical abnormalities on the basis that all of her UTIs are confined to the lower urinary tract. Thus, one could argue that no radiological evaluation is needed, but instead a thorough history should be obtained and any dysfunctional elimination habits addressed as part of the therapeutic course.

13. Studies frequently employed in the initial evaluation of a child with a history of febrile UTIs include all except:

   (a) Intravenous pyelography
   (b) Renal and bladder ultrasound
   (c) Contrast voiding cystourethrogram in boys
   (d) Direct radionuclide cystography in girls
   (e) DMSA renal scintigraphy

Answer: (a)   Intravenous pyelography has no role in the evaluation of the child with UTI. Other imaging protocols, including the standard combination of cystography and sonography, or the recent "top-down" approach that obtains early DMSA renal scans as the first-line evaluation tool, are more appropriate for evaluating.

14. All of the following statements concerning DMSA radionuclide renal scans are true except:

    (a) Transient acute pyelonephritic changes may persist up to 2 months after the initial episode
    (b) Renal scarring on DMSA scans appears as focal or generalized areas of cortical contraction
    (c) Ultrasonography is as accurate as DMSA renal scans in detecting areas of pyelonephritic scarring
    (d) Changes associated with acute pyelonephritis on DMSA renal scans appear as areas of decreased isotope uptake and intact renal cortex without renal volume loss
    (e) DMSA scintigraphy is useful in detecting acute pyelonephritis in children performing clean intermittent catheterization (CIC)

    Answer: (c) Several comparative studies, including one in an experimental model in the piglet, have shown that sonography is half as sensitive as DMSA renal scans for the detection of acute pyelonephritis.

15. Which of the following children requires antimicrobial prophylaxis:

    (a) A 16-year-old myelodysplastic girl without VUR on clean intermittent catheterization and positive urine cultures
    (b) An 8-year-old girl without VUR with three culture documented afebrile UTIs within 18 months
    (c) A 2-year-old uncircumcised boy with a positive urine culture obtained by collection bag
    (d) A 7-year-old girl with surgically corrected VUR and a postoperative isocystogram demonstrating no VUR
    (e) A 5-year-old girl with recurrent febrile UTIs and resolved VUR

    Answer: (e) Regardless of the reflux status, the child in (e) is at greatest risk for acquired renal cortical scarring and thus deserves preventive measures.

16. All of the following regarding the treatment of acute urinary infection is true except:

    (a) A 7-year-old with fevers to 102°F should receive 1–2 days of intramuscular Ceftriaxone to begin therapy
    (b) A 2-month-old girl with a culture documented febrile UTI may be managed on an outpatient basis with oral antibiotics
    (c) Oral antibiotic therapy for acute cystitis should be followed by antibiotic prophylaxis in children <5 years of age until evaluation is completed
    (d) Acute cystitis rarely requires >5 days of oral antibiotics
    (e) Prompt treatment of acute urinary infection in infants is critical in preventing the formation of renal scarring

    Answer: (b) An infant of this age should be managed initially with intravenous antibiotics.

Fungal, parasitic, and other inflammatory diseases of the genitourinary tract

8

Ilene Wong and William A Kennedy II

---

1. What quantity (threshold in cfu/ml) will diagnose true candiduria on suprapubic tap and straight catheterization?

Suprapubic tap	Straight catheterization
(a) Any number of cfu/ml	Any number of cfu/ml
(b) Any number of cfu/ml	>10,000 cfu/ml
(c) >1000 cfu/ml	>20,000 cfu/ml
(d) >10,000 cfu/ml	>15,000 cfu/ml
(e) >10,000 cfu/ml	>100,000 cfu/ml

Answer: (d) The diagnosis of candiduria is frequently complicated by contamination of specimens and the rapid growth of organisms in urine. Kozinn et al[1] have shown colony counts of >10,000 cfu/ml to be associated with clinical infection for suprapubic tap. Wise et al[2] showed that >15,000 cfu/ml signifies true candiduria in straight catheterized females, while a threshold of >100,000 is used to determine candiduria in patients with an indwelling catheter.

2. You are counseling the parents of a 4-month-old child with systemic candidiasis on the potential risks of treatment. Which of the following statements about the treatment of systemic candidiasis with amphotericin B are false?

   (a) Amphotericin B can be nephrotoxic

   (b) Side-effects can include fever and general malaise
   (c) Creatinine should be checked only at the end of therapy
   (d) Peak and trough values of amphotericin B should be two times the minimum inhibitory concentration (MIC) and one time the MIC, respectively
   (e) The treatment course is often required for several weeks

Answer: (c) Amphotericin B treatment carries with it a significant risk of nephrotoxicity, requiring creatinine monitoring every other day. Goal peak and trough levels to minimize toxic side-effects are twice the MIC and one time the MIC. Side-effects include fever, nausea and vomiting as well as generalized malaise. Amphotericin B treatment duration is variable and dependent on the extent of disease.

3. A 7-year-old girl/status post-bone marrow transplant presents with hematuria and dysuria. A CT scan reveals a large fungus ball in her renal pelvis. Urine cultures reveal aspergillosis. What is the next recommended treatment?

   (a) Nephrectomy
   (b) Intravenous fluconazole
   (c) Percutaneous nephrostomy
   (d) Percutaneous nephrostomy followed by amphotericin B irrigation
   (e) Oral fluconazole

Answer: (d) The optimal treatment of a patient with an isolated fungal ball without systemic sepsis is amphotericin B irrigation through a percutaneous nephrostomy tube. Surgical or percutaneous removal of the fungus ball may be required if this fails. If invasive aspergillosis is expected, intravenous amphotericin B is recommended.

4. The radiographic appearance of renal coccydiomycosis is similar to:

(a) Schistosomiasis
(b) Tuberculosis
(c) Renal cell carcinoma
(d) Xanthogranulomatous pyelonephritis
(e) Angiomyolipoma

Answer: (b)   Renal coccydiomycosis is often mistaken for renal tuberculosis in its radiographic appearance, with infundibular stenoses, blunted or sloughed calyces and calcified granulomas frequently seen. Typically the organism is limited to the cortex, presenting with miliary granulomas and microabscesses.

5. Which of the following is *not* one of the sequelae of schistosomiasis infection?

(a) Hematuria
(b) Vesicoureteral reflux
(c) Bladder outlet obstruction
(d) Bladder calculi
(e) Transitional cell carcinoma

Answer: (e)   Schistosomiasis can have widespread genitourinary effects. Acute infection can cause hematuria severe enough to lead to anemia. The inactive infection state, characterized by infiltrative fibrosis, can cause a wide range of lower urinary tract pathology including hydronephrosis, bladder outlet obstruction and vesicoureteral reflux. Complications of urinary stasis, including urinary tract infections, bladder calculi and squamous metaplasia leading to squamous cell carcinoma, can also occur.

6. Which of the following are useful in the diagnosis of echinococcal infections of the urinary system:

(a) The recovery of daughter cysts in the urine
(b) Identification of parasite in urine and feces
(c) Serum enzyme-linked immunosorbent assay (ELISA)
(d) (a) and (c)
(e) (b) and (c)
(f) (a), (b) and (c)

Answer: (d) Echinococcal infections in humans occur during an intermediate stage in the parasitic life cycle. Thus, diagnosis can only be made through the identification of scolices or daughter cysts in the urine rather than by visualization of the parasite itself. Serum ELISA assays can also be used to identify echinococcal infections; however, their increased sensitivity is offset by the possibility of false-positive reactions with other parasites.

7. A 5-year-old human immunodeficiency virus (HIV)-positive girl presents with gross hematuria, dysuria and urge incontinence. Urine cultures at the time are negative. Ultrasound of the bladder shows a diffusely thickened bladder wall. Urine immunofluorescence is positive for adenovirus antigen. What is the next step in treatment?

(a) Aggressive hydration
(b) Cystoscopy and bladder biopsy
(c) Oral fluconazole
(d) Oral corticosteroid therapy
(e) Chemical fulguration with formalin

Answer: (a)   Adenovirus types 11 and 21 are the most common cause of viral cystitis, which has a higher incidence in immunocompromised patients. These infections are usually self-limited and can be treated with fluid resuscitation; resolution of sonographic bladder wall thickening typically occurs in 2–3 weeks.

8. An 8-year-old boy presents with 2 days of gradually worsening left scrotal pain. He is afebrile and a urinalysis is negative. Doppler ultrasound of the scrotum reveals normal flow to bilateral testes and a left hydrocele. He has a history of dysfunctional voiding. What is the most likely etiology for his pain?

   (a) Ectopic ureter draining to the vas deferens
   (b) Torsion of the appendix testis
   (c) Hematogenous spread from a systemic infection
   (d) Retrograde passage of urine from the ejaculatory ducts
   (e) Direct extension from a previous bout of orchitis

   Answer: (d)   Epididymitis can be caused by an infectious agent or chemical irritants. However, Megalli et al[3] have also theorized that retrograde passage of sterile urine from the ejaculatory ducts may cause inflammation. Bukowski et al[4] further suggested that a dysfunctional voiding pattern may cause retrograde flow through due to external sphincter spasm. This is the most likely etiology in a patient who presents with no signs of systemic infection and a sterile urine specimen.

9. Malacoplakia is thought to be caused by:

   (a) An immunoglobin G (IgG) deficiency
   (b) Abnormal macrophage function
   (c) Obstruction by Michaelis-Gutman bodies
   (d) Chronic staphylococcal infections
   (e) Lymphocyte overactivity

   Answer: (b)   Malacoplakia is a benign granulomatous condition thought to be caused by defective digestion by abnormal macrophages. Its histologic appearance is characterized by Michaelis-Gutman bodies, which are "owl-eye" inclusions in the cytoplasm.

10. The physical exam of a child with idiopathic scrotal edema is best aided by:

   (a) Digital rectal exam
   (b) Manipulating the testis into the superficial inguinal pouch for diagnostic palpation
   (c) Evaluation of the contralateral testicle
   (d) Close evaluation of the penis, including retraction of the foreskin
   (e) Palpation of the vas deferens

   Answer: (b)   Characterized by edema confined to the superficial layers of the scrotum in an afebrile child with normal urinalysis, idiopathic scrotal edema is typically self-limiting. Though scrotal ultrasound is often performed, diagnostic palpation after manipulating the testis into the superficial inguinal pouch will normally reveal a nontender and normal testis. Rectal exam and palpation of the vas deferens are nondiagnostic, and the penis is rarely involved.

11. Which of the following are *not* part of the treatment of nonspecific vulvovaginitis?

   (a) Promoting the use of loose-fitting undergarments
   (b) Avoidance of bubble-baths
   (c) Empiric treatment with PO tetracycline
   (d) Examination and identification of vaginal foreign objects
   (e) Emphasizing good handwashing techniques

   Answer: (c)   The treatment of nonspecific vulvovaginitis is typically geared towards reducing risk factors including poor hygiene, use of chemical irritants, presence of foreign objects (including toilet paper) and promoting drying of the vulva by wearing loose-fitting underwear. Treatment of vulvovaginitis with a specific cultured organism is dependent on the species isolated.

References

1. Kozinn PJ, Taschdjian CL, Goldberg PK et al. Advances in the diagnosis of renal candidiasis. J Urol 1978; 119: 184–7.

2. Wise GJ, Goldberg P, Kozinn PJ. Genitourinary candidiasis: diagnosis and treatment. J Urol 1976; 116: 778–80.

3. Megalli M, Gursel E, Lattimer JK. Reflux of urine into ejaculatory ducts as a cause of recurring epididymitis in children. J Urol 1972; 108: 978–9.

4. Bukowski TP, Lewis AG, Reeves D et al. Epididymitis in older boys: dysfunctional voiding as an etiology. J Urol 1995; 154: 762–5.

Pain management for the pediatric patient

9

Jason W Anast and Paul F Austin
(Based on chapter written by Stephen C Brown and Patricia A McGrath)

1. Which of the following is a valid method of assessing pain intensity in a child?

    (a) Patient-reported questionnaire
    (b) Parent-reported checklist of presumed pain-related behaviors
    (c) Pain index based on patient heart rate and blood pressure
    (d) (a) and (b)
    (e) All of the above

    Answer: (d)   Multiple validated scales exist to measure pain in children. Behavioral scale checklists that measure presumed pain behaviors such as crying, limb rigidity, or facial grimacing have been shown to accurately measure acute postoperative pain. Additionally, self-reported pain scales accurately reflect the child's true level of pain. Although physiologic measures such as heart rate and blood pressure provide insight into the level of distress in children, presently there are no valid physiologic pain scales in children.

2. Which of the following medications does *not* have a beneficial effect on pain?

    (a) Gabapentin
    (b) Diclofenac
    (c) Fluoxetine
    (d) Prednisone
    (e) Amitriptyline

    Answer: (c)   Gabapentin is an anticonvulsant which can be effective for treating neuropathic pain. Diclofenac is an anti-inflammatory drug. Prednisone is a corticosteroid which can improve pain due to nerve compression or metastatic disease. Amitriptyline is an antidepressant which can effectively treat neuropathic pain after 1–2 weeks of therapy. Selective serotonin reuptake inhibitors such as fluoxetine are useful for treating depression but have not been shown to improve pain in children.

3. Which of the following regimens is *not* a recommended method for controlling acute postoperative pain in children?

    (a) Intravenous fentanyl
    (b) Intravenous meperidine
    (c) Oral ibuprofen
    (d) Rectal acetaminophen
    (e) Patient-controlled administration of intravenous hydromorphone

    Answer: (a)   In general, the oral route should be utilized to administer pain medications since it avoids the additional pain of intravenous, intramuscular administration. The intramuscular route should be avoided in general because it is often painful and does not deliver reliable dosages. Intravenous fentanyl should not be used for treating acute postoperative pain due to the high risk of respiratory depression or arrest.

4. When performing an inguinal nerve block on an 8 kg child, what is the maximum volume of 0.5% bupivicaine that should be used?

    (a) 2 ml
    (b) 4 ml

(c) 6 ml

(d) 8 ml

(e) 16 ml

Answer: (a) The maximum dose of bupivacaine should not exceed 1.25 mg/kg when performing ilioinguinal block in children <15 kg in weight.[1] For 0.5% bupivicaine, this is equivalent to 0.25 ml/kg, or 2 ml in an 8 kg child.

5. Which of the following statements about the penile block is *not* true?

(a) The targeted nerves run deep to Scarpa's fascia

(b) The penile block provides equivalent anesthesia as the subcutaneous penile ring block

(c) The needle is inserted in the subpubic region just lateral to the midline

(d) The penile ring block is an easily learned technique

(e) Rare complications of penile block include penile ischemia, excessive bleeding, and abscess

Answer: (b) The penile block is a safe and simple anesthetic method for penile surgery. In a prospective study, it was shown that penile block resulted in less pain and less postoperative pain medication than subcutaneous ring block.[2]

References

1. Smith T, Morati P, Wulf H. Smaller children have greater bupivacaine plasma concentration after ilioinguinal block. Br J Anaesth 1996; 76: 452–5.
2. Holder KJ, Peutrell JM, Weir PM. Regional anaesthesia for circumcision. Subcutaneous ring block of the penis and subpubic penile block compared. Eur J Anaesthesiol 1997; 14: 495–8.

Office pediatric urology 10

Kara Saperston, Patrick Cartwright, and Brent Snow

(Based on chapter written by Patrick Cartwright, Timothy Masterson, and Brent Snow)

1. By what age does 95% of physiologic phimosis most commonly resolve?

   (a) 1–2 years of age
   (b) 3–5 years of age
   (c) 6–7 years of age
   (d) 8–9 years of age

   Answer: (b) The physiologic adherence of the preputial attachments to the glans resolves spontaneously around 3–5 years of age. While most texts agree on this age range, Oster performed a longitudinal study that showed some boys will continue to resolve their physiologic phimosis when they are as old as 10 or 11 years of age.[1]

2. The recommended treatment for phimosis includes all of the following except:

   (a) Circumcision
   (b) Use of topical corticosteroids
   (c) Forceful separation of the inner prepuce and glans penis
   (d) Watchful waiting

   Answer: (c) Forceful separation of foreskin adhesions is not recommended because of pain and trauma to the patient; gentle proximal traction of the foreskin may enable one to differentiate between normal and abnormal phimosis. Circumcision is recommended for pathologic phimosis, and topical steroids and watchful waiting may aid in physiologic phimosis.

3. Non-neonatal circumcision is most commonly performed because of:

   (a) Balanoposthitis
   (b) Phimosis
   (c) Urinary tract infections (UTIs)
   (d) Zipper trauma

   Answer: (b) Non-neonatal circumcision is most commonly performed because of phimosis; while balanoposthitis and zipper trauma are causes for circumcision they are not the most common cause. UTIs in uncircumcised males appear to be more common only in the first 6 months of life; after 1 year of age it is felt the risk for UTIs diminishes significantly and does not warrant circumcision.

4. A finding on voiding cystourethrogram (VCUG) consistent with urethral prolapse is:

   (a) Narrow distal urethra
   (b) Wide bladder neck
   (c) Vaginal voiding
   (d) Inability to void

   Answer: (a) Urethral prolapse appears as a doughnut-shaped mass protruding at the vulva. It is usually diagnosed based on appearance of the lesions. At times it is confirmed by placing a catheter in the urethra. Imaging is not necessary but a narrow distal urethra has been seen on VCUG.

5. Asymptomatic labial adherence is best treated with:

   (a) Separation in the operating room
   (b) EMLA cream and gentle blunt separation in the office
   (c) Estrogen cream
   (d) Observation

   Answer: (d) Labial adherence is described as the midline fusion of the labia minora.

Its peak incidence is between birth and 2 years, and again around 6–7 years of age. Treatment is not routinely required and the adhesions should lyse spontaneously, but separation in the operating room, the office or the use of estrogen cream have been tried when there are associated symptoms.

6. Gartner's duct cysts in the newborn period are:

(a) Remnants of nonfused portions of the Müllerian ducts
(b) Remnants of the urogenital sinus
(c) Posterior
(d) Rudimentary portions of the Wolffian duct

Answer: (d) Gartner's duct is the distal rudimentary portion of the Wolffian duct in girls. They usually regress but if persistent they are found on the anterolateral walls of the vagina. They present as a perivaginal mass in infants, and can be large enough to protrude and fill the vagina.

7. Yeast infections, other than diaper rash, in 4- and 5-year-old girls are caused by:

(a) Depressed cellular immunity
(b) Alkaline vaginal pH
(c) Prophylactic antibiotics
(d) A warm, moist environment

Answer: (a) Yeast infections are more common in adult females than in prepubertal girls. The alkaline vaginal pH of childhood is hostile to yeast. Most yeast vaginitis is caused by *Candida albicans*, and is secondary to host factors such as depressed cellular immunity or broad-spectrum antibiotics.

8. Helpful studies in persistent microscopic hematuria include:

(a) Calcium:creatinine ratio

(b) Nuclear medicine renal scan
(c) Renal ultrasound
(d) Hemoglobin electrophoresis

Answer: (c) All of the above except for nuclear medicine renal scan aid in assessing for hypercalciuria. A calcium:creatinine ratio with help identify idiopathic calciuria, a renal ultrasound will rule out a mass in the kidney or stones, and hemoglobin electrophoresis will rule out sickle-cell trait or disease.

9. Glomerular source of hematuria is often:

(a) Bright red and normal morphology on microscopic exam
(b) Cola-colored urine
(c) Absence of red blood cells (RBCs) on microscopic exam
(d) Associated with flank pain

Answer: (b) Glomerular source hematuria is often cola or tea colored; bright red and normal morphology suggests the urinary tract. The absence of RBCs on micro but the positive dipstick indicates myoglobinuria or hemoglobinuria. Flank pain often insinuates obstructive causes either from gross hemorrhage or clot.

10. Idiopathic urethrorrhagia in prepubertal boys presents with all but:

(a) 30% have dysuria
(b) Blood spotting between voiding
(c) Normal ultrasound (US) and VCUG
(d) Urinalysis (UA) with RBCs in 57% of patients
(e) Resolution with antibiotics

Answer: (e) Idiopathic urethrorrhagia is seen in prepubertal boys who present with blood spotting in their underwear between voiding. A review at the University of Utah showed 30% had dysuria, 57% had UA with RBCs, a normal US and VCUG. The symptoms would range from a few weeks to 3 years, and resolved spontaneously without antibiotics.

Reference

1. Oster J. Further fate of the foreskin: incidence of preputial adhesions, phimosis and smegma among Danish schoolboys. Arch Dis Child 1968; 43: 200–3.

Principles of minimally invasive surgery

11

Walid Farhat and Pasquale Casale

1. When performing laparoscopic pediatric urological procedure, necessary intraoperative monitoring should include all of the following except:

    (a) Routine electrocardiogram
    (b) Noninvasive blood pressure
    (c) Arterial lines
    (d) Temperature
    (e) Inspired oxygen concentration

    Answer: (c) Although end-tidal CO_2 may not accurately reflect arterial CO_2 tension, its use is helpful to plan appropriate ventilation strategies. On the other hand, in infants and children with respiratory pathology, capillary or arterial blood gas analysis might be indicated to accurately measure CO_2 tension.

2. Trendelenburg position during laparoscopy will cause all of the following except:

    (a) Increased heart rate
    (b) Decreased vascular resistance
    (c) Decreased mean arterial pressure
    (d) Decreased cardiac output

    Answer: (b) Patient positioning during laparoscopic surgery is capable of affecting and further potentiating the impact of gas insufflation. For instance, a Trendelenburg position during laparoscopy will increase the heart rate and vascular resistance while decreasing mean arterial pressure and cardiac output.

3. Decreased urine output during laparoscopic surgery is secondary to:

    (a) Decreased renal vascular resistance
    (b) Decreased cardiac output
    (c) Ureteral compression
    (d) Decreased renal blood flow
    (e) None of the above

    Answer: (d) The renal effects occur secondary to gas insufflation manifested by decreased glomerular filtration rate and urine output. Animal studies have shown that gas insufflation causes renal vein compression inducing decreased renal blood flow; urine output drops and diminished creatinine clearance.

4. Currently, the following are contraindications to laparoscopy except for:

    (a) Cardiopulmonary morbidity
    (b) Uncorrected coagulopathy
    (c) Sepsis
    (d) Small bowel obstruction
    (e) Malignant kidney tumor

    Answer: (d) Contraindications to laparoscopy in infants, children, and adolescents are the same as for any other surgical procedure, except for evidence of limited lung reserve function, which may be considered as relative contraindications. If the patients is septic, in shock, or exhibits a coagulopathy, these should be corrected before surgery is contemplated. If surgery is deemed essential under these circumstances, then it probably should be performed open. Furthermore, although laparoscopy may play a role in the staging of malignant pediatric abdominal tumors such as Wilms or neuroblastoma, its role in the management of these tumors has yet to be defined.

5. The boundaries of the retroperitoneal space are the following except for:

    (a) Posteriorly and laterally: the transversalis and quadratus lumborum muscles
    (b) Anteriorly: the mobile posterior parietal peritoneum and its contents
    (c) Superiorly: the diaphragm
    (d) Inferiorly: contiguous with the extraperitoneal portions of the pelvis
    (e) None of the above

    Answer: (a)   An understanding of the retroperitoneal surgical anatomy is mandatory before embarking on retroperitoneoscopic surgery. Posteriorly and laterally: the paraspinal, psoas, and quadratus lumborum muscles, which are anatomically, fixed structures.
    Anteriorly: the mobile posterior parietal peritoneum and its contents.
    Superiorly: the diaphragm.
    Inferiorly: contiguous with the extraperitoneal portions of the pelvis.

6. When vascular injury occurs during laparoscopic procedure:

    (a) Immediate removal of the trocars and conversion to open exploration is undertaken
    (b) It may be unnoticed, thus may not need any intervention
    (c) When minor such as tear of gonadal vessels, traction on the kidney posteriorly may help stop the bleeding
    (d) Routine inspection of the electrocautery instruments prior to any laparoscopic procedure is mandatory
    (e) None of the above

    Answer: (d)   The hallmark features of vascular injuries include either bloody return from the injury site or rapid deterioration of the hemodynamic status of the patient. Once extensive vascular injury is suspected, the trocar should be left in place and an open exploration should be performed. However, if minor vascular injury is encountered during dissection, such as laceration to the gonadal vessels or adrenal vessels, hemostasis should be maintained with traction anteriorly on the kidney, thus stretching those vessels, and continually observing and maintaining normal patient's vital signs. On the other hand, to decrease the risk of injury while dissecting, in addition to paramount care while dissecting, it is mandatory that there is a thorough understanding of the anatomy, equipment, and meticulous attention to details.

7. During laparoscopic procedures:

    (a) Patient positioning in the pediatric patient rarely affects the impact of gas insufflation
    (b) Trendelenburg position during laparoscopy will increase heart rate and vascular resistance
    (c) Reverse Trendelenburg position increases mean arterial pressure and cardiac output
    (d) Left flank positioning accentuates impaired venous return more than the right flank position
    (e) None of the above

    Answer: (d)   Trendelenburg position during laparoscopy will increase heart rate and vascular resistance while decreasing mean arterial pressure and cardiac output, while the opposite effect is seen in a reverse Trendelenburg position. Furthermore, flank positioning especially with the kidney rest up and patient flexed will accentuate impaired venous return and increase cardiac strain. Particularly, the left lateral decibitus position produces far more significant hemodynamic and respiratory changes than the right flank position.

8. The advantages of retroperitoneal approach are true all except:

    (a) The technique mimics the open urological surgical procedure

(b) It provides direct approach to the organs of the genitourinary tract

(c) Colon or splenic injuries do not occur in this approach

(d) Facilitates the view of the posterior surface of the kidney, hence rapid access to the renal hilum

(e) Previous transperitoneal surgery does not preclude retroperitoneoscopy

Answer: (c) Retroperitoneoscopy provides direct approach to the organs of the genitourinary tract, and requires less dissection to the colon or the spleen to expose the kidneys and adrenals. Furthermore, previous transperitoneal surgery does not preclude retroperitoneoscopy. Finally, it facilitates the view of the posterior surface of the kidney and hence rapid access to the renal hilum. On the other hand, the disadvantages of retroperitoneal laparoscopy are that manipulation of instruments may be initially difficult due to a restrictive working space.

9. When performing a retroperitoneal laparoscopic procedure, all of the following are correct except:

(a) Access may be achieved by the closed technique

(b) Veress needle may rarely cause injury to the great vessels

(c) Insertion of the primary trocar far medially may result in peritoneal entry or colon injury

(d) Initial dissection of the kidney anteriorly is undertaken

(e) None of the above

Answer: (c) Access to the retroperitoneum is preferably achieved by the open (Hasson) technique, which provides visual guidance to the correct retroperitoneal space. As children have a small retroperitoneal space – and close proximity between the abdominal wall and the major vessels, which are primarily retroperitoneal – the closed technique is not recommended. In addition, since there is no actual pre-existing retroperitoneal space, placement of Veress needle is not accurate and may inadvertently be positioned deep in the retroperitoneum causing either injury to the great vessels or pneumoperitoneum, thereby complicating the procedure.

10. Relative contraindications to a retroperitoneal approach are all the following except:

(a) Prior retroperitoneal scar (kidney surgery, kidney biopsy or pyeloplasty)

(b) Previous infectious or inflammatory retroperitoneal process

(c) Cardiopulmonary morbidity

(d) Uncorrected coagulopathy

(e) Sepsis

Answer: (b) Contraindications to laparoscopy in infants, children, and adolescents are the same as for any other surgical procedure, except for evidence of limited lung reserve function, which may be considered as relative contraindications. If the patient is septic, in shock, or exhibits a coagulopathy, these should be corrected before surgery is contemplated. If surgery is deemed essential under these circumstances, then it probably should be performed open.

Absolute contraindications: cardiopulmonary morbidity; uncorrected coagulopathy; sepsis.

Relative contraindications: prior retroperitoneal scar (kidney surgery, kidney biopsy or pyeloplasty); previous infectious or inflammatory retroperitoneal process (xanthogranulomatous pyelonephritis) except for experienced surgeons in this approach.

Pediatric fluid management 12

Paul F Austin

(Based on chapter written by James M Robertson)

1. The daily maintenance fluid requirement for a 9 kg infant is:

   (a) 600 ml/day
   (b) 700 ml/day
   (c) 800 ml/day
   (d) 900 ml/day
   (e) 1000 ml/day

   Answer: (d)   Metabolism parallels the utilization of water. Holliday and Segar found that infants and children weighing 0–10 kg require 100 cal/kg/day. Because 1 cal of energy requires a net consumption of 1 ml of water, the answer is 9 kg × 100 ml/kg/day = 900 ml/day.[1]

2. The hourly maintenance fluid requirement of this same 9 kg infant is:

   (a) 25 ml/h
   (b) 30 ml/h
   (c) 33 ml/h
   (d) 36 ml/h
   (e) 42 ml/h

   Answer: (d)   Hourly maintenance fluid requirements can be stratified by the following patient weights: 4 ml/kg/h for 0–10 kg; 40 ml/h + 2 ml/kg/h per kg for 11–20 kg; 60 ml/h + 1 ml/kg/h per kg >20 kg. In the following example, the 9 kg infant would require 9 kg × 4 ml/kg/h = 36 ml/h.

3. The daily maintenance fluid requirement for a 35 kg child is:

   (a) 1600 ml/day
   (b) 1700 ml/day
   (c) 1800 ml/day
   (d) 1900 ml/day
   (e) 2000 ml/day

   Answer: (c)   Daily maintenance fluid requirements can be stratified by the following patient weights: 100 ml/kg/day for 0–10 kg; 1000 ml/day + 50 ml/kg/day per kg for 11–20 kg; 1500 ml/day + 20 ml/kg/day per kg >20 kg. In the following example, the 35 kg infant would require 1500 ml/day + (15 kg × 20 ml/kg/h) = 1800 ml/day.

4. The hourly maintenance fluid requirement of a 40 kg child is:

   (a) 75 ml/h
   (b) 80 ml/h
   (c) 85 ml/h
   (d) 90 ml/h
   (e) 95 ml/h

   Answer: (b)   Hourly maintenance fluid requirements can be stratified by the following patient weights: 4 ml/kg/h for 0–10 kg; 40 ml/h + 2 ml/kg/h per kg for 11–20 kg; 60 ml/h + 1 ml/kg/h per kg >20 kg. In the following example, the 40 kg child would require 60 ml + (20 kg × 1 ml/kg/h) = 80 ml/h.

5. Which of the following statements is *not* true?

   (a) Potassium is the major cation in the intracellular space
   (b) Sodium is the major cation in the extracellular space

    (c) Major losses of sodium, potassium, and chloride occur via the kidney

    (d) Urine concentrating ability is impaired at birth

    (e) Premature infants have low renal sodium loss

Answer: (e)   Premature infants, in particular, have high intestinal and renal sodium losses. Sodium reabsorption is poor and intrarenal gradients of NaCl are not yet developed. Urine-concentrating ability is impaired, and salt and water losses are great.

6. The electrolyte and glucose requirements for a 9 kg infant are:

    (a) 27 mEq Na$^+$/day, 18 mEq K$^+$/day, 36 g glucose/day

    (b) 18 mEq Na$^+$/day, 9 mEq K$^+$/day, 27 g glucose/day

    (c) 27 mEq Na$^+$/day, 9 mEq K$^+$/day, 27 g glucose/day

    (d) 18 mEq Na$^+$/day, 12 mEq K$^+$/day, 36 g glucose/day

    (e) 18 mEq Na$^+$/day, 12 mEq K$^+$/day, 27 g glucose/day

Answer: (a)   Holliday and Seger observed that human milk contained the minimal electrolyte requirements for infants, and electrolyte requirements for infants were 3.0 mEq/100 cal/day for sodium and 2.0 mEq/100 cal/day for both potassium and chloride. Glucose requirements are 25 g/100 cal. For a 9 kg infant, their daily caloric requirement is 100 cal/kg/day or 9 kg×100 cal/kg/day=900 cal/day. Subsequently a 9 kg infant would require supplementation with 27 mEq Na$^+$/day, 18 mEq K$^+$/day, 36 g glucose/day.[1]

7. With regard to fluid compartments in the newborn:

    (a) Total body water is lowest in premature infants

    (b) The extracellular fluid is the largest compartment of the total body water

    (c) Intravascular volume is low and increases with age

    (d) Intracellular fluid is high and decreases with age

    (e) Intracellular fluid includes the interstitial volume and transcellular fluid

Answer: (b)   Total body water (TBW) is highest in the preterm infant at 80% body weight. By term, TBW has decreased to 70–75% and continues to fall during the immediate postnatal period to 60–65% during the latter part of the first year of life. The extracellular fluid compartment comprises the bulk of the TBW and parallels this decrease by percent body weight with maturity: 60% body weight in the premature infant; 45% in the term infant; and 30% in the adolescent. Intravascular volume (ml/kg) is highest in premature infants and diminishes with age. Intracellular fluid is the only fluid compartment which increases with age based on percent body weight. The interstitial volume and transcellular fluid are divisions of the extracellular fluid compartment.

8. Which of the following statements regarding intravenous fluids is false:

    (a) Hypotonic fluids are appropriate for maintenance of TBW and electrolyte balance when given in amounts reflective of normal physiologic requirements

    (b) Isotonic fluids that most closely match serum and plasma osmolarity in children are 270–290 mOsm/kg

    (c) Half normal saline is a hypotonic fluid

    (d) Dextrose is a transient osmole and once metabolized the osmolarity of the solution diminishes

    (e) Isotonic solutions are solutions with an osmolarity that is comparable to that of intracellular fluid but greater than that of the extracellular fluid compartment

Answer: (e)   Ideally, there is no change in the intracellular and extracellular osmolar gradient.

Isotonic solutions are solutions with an osmolarity that is comparable to that of the extracellular fluid as well as the intracellular fluid compartment.

9. Which of the following statements regarding intraoperative fluid therapy is false:

   (a) Isotonic fluids are used intraoperatively at rates necessary to maintain intravascular volume and adequate perfusion
   (b) Relative to awake resting requirements, there is an increased need for sodium replacement intraoperatively due to excess free water retention from the increased antidiuretic hormone (ADH) that is stimulated from the stress of surgery
   (c) Lactated Ringer's solution is the most common isotonic fluid which is used for ongoing replacement of intraoperative fluid losses
   (d) 5% dextrose solution is acceptable for fluid replacement intraoperatively
   (e) Blood loss may be replaced in a one-to-one ratio with colloid or three- to fourfold with crystalloid

Answer: (d) The administration of dextrose to pediatric patients under anesthesia is debatable and although intraoperative stress increases blood sugar, the risk of preoperative hypoglycemia due to fasting is estimated at 1–2%. The use of 5% dextrose solution intraoperatively has been associated with hyperglycemia and should not be used for fluid replacement.

10. Which of the following statements regarding postoperative fluid therapy is false:

   (a) The allowable blood loss may be calculated by knowing the patient's weight, estimated blood volume, initial hemoglobin, and minimal allowable hemoglobin
   (b) Hyperkalemia and hypercalcemia with transfusion are dependent on the rate of transfusion
   (c) Dilution with saline is advised for slow infusions, since calcium in lactated Ringer's solution may promote microaggregate formation in the intravenous line
   (d) Fluid losses should be replaced with isotonic fluids
   (e) Intravenous fluid therapy in the postoperative period is an extension of intraoperative therapy, and changes in fluid and electrolyte homeostasis are still under the influence of surgical or traumatic stress

Answer: (b) Sodium citrate is added to packed red blood cells (PRBCs) and fresh frozen plasma to chelate calcium and prevent clotting. Citrate administered with these blood products may therefore lead to hypocalcemia. PRBCs contain a high level of potassium which may increase with storage and therefore can lead to hyperkalemia.

Reference

1. Holliday MA, Segar WE. The maintenance need for water in parenteral fluid therapy. Pediatrics 1957; 19: 823–32.

Embryology of adrenal, kidney, ureteral development, renal vasculature, and gonads

Steven E Lerman, Irene M McAleer, and George W Kaplan

---

1. There are three sets of kidneys that develop in mammals during embryogenesis. Which of these primitive kidneys do not function during development?

   (a) Pronephros
   (b) Mesonephros
   (c) Metanephric mass
   (d) All of the primitive kidneys function at some time, however brief, during mammalian development

   Answer: (a)   The pronephros (pronephroi – plural) develops during the first 21 days of development and does not function in mammals but is analogous to the kidney in primitive fish. The other primitive developing kidneys do function during development; the pronephric ducts are necessary for formation of the mesonephros. (Ch 19, page 285)

2. Autosomic recessive polycystic kidney disease (ARPKD) is a rare inherited disorder with the abnormal renal configuration due to:

   (a) Abnormal branching of the cystic duct and cyst formation in other parts of the renal tubules
   (b) Abnormal formation of the distal convoluted tubule
   (c) Enlargement of the cystic ducts

   (d) Early obstruction of tubules from blockage of the developing ureteral bud

   Answer: (c)   The cysts in ARPKD are due to enlargement of the cystic ducts. Also associated is periportal hepatic fibrosis. The cysts in ADPKD are due to abnormal branching of the cystic duct and formation of cysts in other parts of the renal tubules (making (a) incorrect). This disorder is much more common than ARPKD. The early obstruction of the renal tubules from faulty development or blockage of the ureteral bud is thought to be responsible for the findings in multicystic dysplastic kidneys (MCDK) (making (d) incorrect). None of these disorders is due to abnormal formation of the distal convoluted tubule (making (b) incorrect). (Ch 19, page 289)

3. Adrenal cortical development in human embryogenesis is noted by the 8th week of gestation and is comprised of:

   (a) Fetal zone, zona glomerulosa, and zona fasciculata
   (b) Primitive zona glomerulosa, fasciculata, and reticularis
   (c) Fetal zone and adrenal cortical cells
   (d) Primitive neural crest cells interspersed with primitive adrenocortical cells

   Answer: (c)   The cortex develops around the 8th week of gestation and is comprised of the rather large central fetal zone and the thin peripheral adrenal cortical cells that are the precursors to the zona glomerulosa, fasciculata and reticularis. The zona glomerulosa and fasiculata develop late in gestation while the zona reticularis will not be apparent until after the 3rd year of life (making (a) and (b) incorrect). The neural crest cells found in the adrenal gland are in the medulla and are not interspersed during development in the cortex of the adrenal (making (d) incorrect). (Ch 14, page 237)

4. The inferior vena cava forms at the level of the renal veins by:

   (a) Merging the right and left subcardinal veins
   (b) Persistence of the right supracardinal vein
   (c) Persistence of the right subcardinal vein
   (d) Persistence of the left supracardinal vein

   Answer: (c) The inferior vena cava is comprised of the right subcardinal vein making up the inferior vena cava from the level of the renal veins and cephalad. The inferior vena cava *below* the renal veins is comprised of the right *supra*cardinal vein (making (b) incorrect). The left supracardinal and the left subcardinal vein systems disappear almost completely, except for the common stem of the left renal vein, left adrenal vein and the left gonadal vein, all comprised of the left subcardinal venous system (making (d) incorrect). There is no merging of the right or left subcardinal systems to create the inferior vena cava (making (a) incorrect). (Ch 19, page 283)

5. Accessory renal arteries are:

   (a) Less common than accessory renal veins
   (b) Result from failure of involution of precursor arteries

   (c) Occur in about 35% of adult kidneys
   (d) Both (b) and (c)

   Answer: (b) Accessory renal arteries are more common than the occurrence of accessory renal veins and are found in about 25% of adult kidneys (making (a), (c) and (d) incorrect). During renal ascent from the pelvis, the developing kidneys receive their vascular supply from those vessels that are closest to them in descent, starting with the common iliacs and ultimately arising from branches off the aorta as the kidneys stop at the adrenal gland area. If the arteries do not involute during the ascent of the kidney, there will be accessory or supernumerary renal arteries (making (b) correct). Ureteral obstruction at the renal pelvis can occur if an inferiorly placed accessory artery is present and crosses over the ureter in the inferior location. (Ch 19, page 283)

6. The posterior cardinal veins form dorsal to the developing kidneys in:

   (a) The mesonephros phase
   (b) The pronephros phase
   (c) The metanephric phase
   (d) The nephrogenic cord phase

   Answer: (a) The postcardinal veins or posterior cardinal veins develop early in vasculature formation to allow return of blood to the heart. They run dorsal to the mesonephros and are the venous supply to the mesonephros (making (a) correct). Eventually the postcardinal veins will disappear except for remnants which will become the root of the azygos vein and the common iliac veins. The subcardinal vein on the left will become the left renal vein to the metanephric tissue and the subcardinal vein meeting the supracardinal vein on the right will be the right renal vein location (making (c) incorrect). The nephrogenic cord is the entire bulk of pronephros, mesonephros and metanephric pluripotential renal tissue, so is correct but is not as specific as the mesonephros (making (d) incorrect). The pronephros forms early in the 4th gestational week and involute before functioning and prior to development of the blood supply of the developing mesonephric tissue (making (b) incorrect). (Ch 19, page 283)

7. The ureteric bud, arising from a bend in the mesonephric duct, pushes into the metanephric blastema, inducing the development of the permanent kidney in the:

   (a) 5th gestational week
   (b) 8th gestational week
   (c) 10th gestational week
   (d) 12th gestational week

   Answer: (a) Early development of the permanent kidney occurs during the 5th gestational week when the ureteric bud meets up with the metanephric mass. By the 6th week the kidney has ascended above the umbilical arteries and by the 8th week the center of the kidney has reached its permanent level just below the adrenal gland (making (b) incorrect). The fetal kidney will start to secrete urine by the 10th gestational week (making (c) incorrect). From the 6th to 20th gestational weeks, the major calices subdivide into the 12 generations of caliceal formation (making (d) incorrect). (Ch 19, page 287)

8. During kidney development, WT1, a Wilms' tumor suppressor gene, is suggested to:

   (a) Make the kidney more resistant to antenatally developing Wilms' tumors
   (b) Not have any role in the development of the permanent kidney
   (c) Cause the ureteral bud to join the metanephric blastema
   (d) Allow the metanephric mass to induce ureteral bud formation

   Answer: (d) Although molecular studies involved deal with laboratory animals, it appears that WT1 is necessary for the metanephric mass to induce the ureteral bud to form probably through regulation of GDNF (glial-cell-line neurotrophic factor). (b) and (c) are incorrect as WT1 appears to be important in the development of the permanent kidney and it is not by inducing the ureteral bud to join with the metanephric blastema. There is no indication, at this time, that WT1 makes the kidney resistant to Wilms' tumor development during the prenatal time period (making (a) incorrect). (Ch 19, page 288)

9. Horseshoe kidneys occur because there is fusion of the lower poles of the developing kidneys and:

   (a) The ascent is arrested by the superior mesenteric artery
   (b) Is fairly common occurring in 1 in 500 people
   (c) Have no higher risk of Wilms' tumor development than the general population
   (d) Both (b) and (c) are correct

   Answer: (b) Horseshoe kidneys occur during the ascent of kidneys but where the two developing metanephric masses come in contact with the lower poles later in development. Horseshoe kidneys are fairly common occurring in 1 in 500 people and also have a 2–8 times higher risk of developing Wilms' tumors than the general population (making (c) and (d) incorrect). The ascent is arrested by the inferior mesenteric artery and not the superior mesenteric artery (making (a) incorrect). (Ch 19, page 289)

10. The adrenal cortex develops as two distinct areas, with the permanent cortex as an outer rind comprised at birth of:

    (a) Zona glomerulosa and zona fasciculata
    (b) Zona glomerulosa, zona fasciculata, and zona reticularis
    (c) Zona fasciculata and zona reticularis

(d) Undifferentiated cortex tissue that will differentiate in the first year of life

Answer: (a) The adrenal cortex develops as a large fetal zone and a small rind permanent adrenal cortex which will become the eventual adult cortex. During late gestation, this thin rind will differentiate into the hormone-producing areas of the zona glomerulosa, producing aldosterone, and zona fasciculata, producing glucocorticoid hormones. The zona reticularis, which will produce the sex or androgen hormones, does not develop until about the third year of life (making (b) and (d) incorrect). (d) is incorrect as there is also a thin rind of the permanent adult cortex tissue around the adrenal gland at birth. (Ch 14, page 237)

11. As part of the fetal hypothalamic–pituitary–adrenal axis, fetal adrenal glucocorticoids stimulate:

(a) The fetal hypothalamus to release corticotrophin-releasing hormone (CRF)
(b) The fetal pituitary to release adrenocorticotrophin (ACTH)
(c) The placenta to release placental CRF
(d) Both (b) and (c) are correct

Answer: (c) The fetal hypothalamic–pituitary–adrenal axis is necessary for the development, differentiation and maturation of vital organ systems such as the lungs, brain and liver which are critical for immediate postnatal survival of the infant. If increased, the fetal glucocorticoids will cause the fetal CRF and fetal pituitary ACTH to be downregulated to decrease the fetal CRF and ACTH (making (a), (b) and (d) incorrect). The fetal adrenal glucocorticoids stimulate the placenta to release CRF causing the fetal adrenal to increase production of the glucocorticoids, thought to be so critical for the transition from fetal to infant life, which may explain why extremely premature infants do not transition well to normal infant life if they are born before normal adrenal development takes place. (Ch 14, page 238)

Extra questions

1. The bladder develops from:

(a) The urogenital sinus
(b) Mesoderm of the anterior abdominal wall
(c) Endoderm
(d) Ureteral buds
(e) All of the above

Answer: (e)

2. Place the following events in correct chronological order:

(a) Pronephros involutes
(b) Urorectal septum descends
(c) Proximal urethra forms
(d) Müllerian ducts form
(e) Wolffian ducts form

    (i) (a), (b), (c), (d), (e)
   (ii) (a), (b), (e), (c), (d)
  (iii) (a), (b), (c), (e), (d)
  (iv) (a), (d), (c), (b), (e)
   (v) (a), (e), (b), (c), (d)

Answer: (v)

3. The fetal gonads begin to differentiate into either a testis or an ovary at approximately which week of gestation?

(a) Week 3
(b) Week 6
(c) Week 9
(d) Week 12
(e) Week 15

Answer: (b)

4. Testicular descent from the abdominal cavity through the inguinal canal and into the

scrotum may be influenced by all of the following except:

(a) Gubernacular guidance
(b) Increased intra-abdominal pressure
(c) Local hormonal factors
(d) The processus vaginalis
(e) Completed development of the vas deferens

Answer: (e)

5. Remnant(s) of the Müllerian duct system is (are):

(a) Appendix testis
(b) Epoopheron
(c) Gartner's duct
(d) (b) and (e)
(e) All of the above

Answer: (a)

Radiologic assessment of the adrenal

15

Karoush Afshar, Douglas H Jamieson, and
Andrew MacNeily

1. All of the following adrenal masses demonstrate high signal intensity on T2-weighted
magnetic resonance imaging (MRI) except
one. Choose the exception:

   (a) Pheochromocytoma
   (b) Acute adrenal hemorrhage
   (c) Neuroblastoma
   (d) Adrenal cyst

   Answer: (b) Fresh blood possesses low
   signal intensity on T2-weighted MRI. After
   liquefaction of the hematoma over several
   weeks, signal intensity increases. All the other
   lesions listed possess bright characteristics on
   T2-weighted MRI.

2. In a case of antenatally diagnosed adrenal
mass, which of the following features on postnatal ultrasounds is against the diagnosis of
neuroblastoma:

   (a) Size >3 cm
   (b) Increase in size on serial ultrasounds
   (c) Development of internal echoes
   (d) Solid homogeneity

   Answer: (c) Development of internal echoes,
   calcifications, or shrinkage suggest resolving
   hematoma. Size >3 cm, solid homogeneous
   mass and increase in size imply neuroblastoma.

3. Which of the following entities represents the
most common neonatal adrenal mass?

   (a) Neuroblastoma

   (b) Adrenal hemorrhage
   (c) Pheochromocytoma
   (d) Ganglioneuroma

   Answer: (b) The most commonly found
   neonatal adrenal mass is an adrenal hemorrhage. These are commonly detected on antenatal maternal fetal ultrasound and are found
   more often on the right-hand side. The latter
   is thought to be secondary to compression
   between the liver and kidney anteriorly, and
   the spine posteriorly.

4. An antenatal ultrasound reveals a 2 cm right
adrenal mass. Postnatally, this is confirmed to
be a 2 cm hyperechoic and septated adrenal
mass. Which of the following represents the
best next step in management?

   (a) Right adrenalectomy
   (b) MRI
   (c) Computerized tomography (CT) scan
   (d) Serial ultrasounds

   Answer: (d) Small hyperechoic adrenal
   lesions detected antenatally, and confirmed
   postnatally, are most commonly adrenal
   hemorrhages. These can be observed with serial
   ultrasounds. Enlargement, or a primarily solid
   appearance, would mandate more aggressive
   imaging and biochemical investigations.

5. A 3 cm solid hyperechoic adrenal lesion is
found incidentally on an ultrasound performed

for abdominal pain in a 4-year-old child. MRI reveals high signal intensity on T1-weighted images and low signal intensity on T2-weighted images. What is the most likely diagnosis?

(a) Pheochromocytoma
(b) Myelolipoma
(c) Adrenal cortical carcinoma
(d) Neuroblastoma

Answer: (b) Myelolipoma is a benign adrenal neoplasm composed of fat and myeloid elements. Typically fat is hyperechoic on ultrasound imaging, exhibits high signal intensity on T1-weighted images and low signal intensity on T2-weighted imaging. The other three malignancies exhibit varying degrees of low intenstity on T1 and high intensity on T2 imaging.

Adrenal tumors and functional consequences

16

Julie Franc-Guimond, Anne-Marie Houle, and Aseem R Shukla

1. Cushing's syndrome is:

   (a) Caused by pituitary hypersecretion of adrenocorticotropic hormone (ACTH)
   (b) Always diagnosed in the presence of hyperparathyroidism, pancreatic-duodenal, and pituitary tumors
   (c) A clinical disorder seen in cases of overproduction of cortisol regardless of the cause
   (d) Observed with catecholamine-secreting tumors
   (e) Observed with several genetic syndromes

   Answer: (c)   Cushing's syndrome is a clinical disorder seen in cases of overproduction of cortisol, as opposed to Cushing's disease which is specifically caused by the pituitary hypersecretion of ACTH. The increased cortisol production leads to protein catabolism, subsequent increased glucose production, and typical symptoms of cortisol excess.

2. Aldosterone secretion is modulated by:

   (a) Plasma estradiol and/or estrone
   (b) Potassium balance, dopamine, and atrial natriuretic peptide
   (c) A low plasma corticotropin-releasing hormone (CRH) level, associated with elevated plasma cortisol concentration
   (d) The secretion of catecholamines and vasoactive intestinal polypeptides
   (e) Androgenic hormones

   Answer: (b)   Aldosterone production from the zona glomerulosa of the adrenal cortex is modulated by the renin-angiotensin system. Aldosterone release may be affected by potassium balance, ACTH, dopamine, and atrial natriuretic peptide.

3. Primary hyperaldosteronism caused by an aldosterone-producing adenoma (APA) is best managed by:

   (a) Bilateral adrenalectomy
   (b) Spironolactone administration
   (c) Potassium supplementation
   (d) Salt restriction
   (e) Unilateral adrenalectomy

   Answer: (e)   An adrenal mass, especially in an individual with hypokalemia and hypertension, raises the suspicion of an APA. Computerized tomography (CT) scanning or magnetic resonance imaging (MRI), and adrenal vein sampling of aldosterone and cortisol when required, confirms an APA that is best managed by a unilateral adrenalectomy.

4. In cases of primary hyperaldosteronism with inconclusive data or equivocal radiographic features, _____ is recommended to differentiate between an adenoma and hyperplasia.

   (a) A therapeutic trial with daily administration of amiloride
   (b) Measurement of plasma adrenal androgens and testosterone
   (c) Pharmacological blockade (alpha and beta) of catecholamine effects and synthesis

(d) Adrenal vein sampling of aldosterone and cortisol

(e) Measurements of elevated plasma estradiol and/or estrone

Answer: (d) When a dexamethasone suppression test and CT or MRI sampling are all equivocal, adrenal vein sampling of aldosterone and cortisol is recommended to differentiate between an adenoma and hyperplasia. Amiloride or spironolactone are appropriate as medical management in cases of bilateral adrenal hyperplasia. Adrenal androgens and testosterone are not measured in this case since aldosterone is the main mineralocorticoid secreted by the adrenal gland.

5. Which conditions lead to reduced "effective" circulating blood volume?

   (a) Congestive heart failure (CHF), hepatic cirrhosis, nephrotic syndrome
   (b) Renovascular disorders, coarctation of the aorta, renin-secreting tumors
   (c) Gitelman's syndrome, Bartter's syndrome
   (d) Diuretic use, pseudohypoaldosteronism Type I
   (e) Emotional stress, physical activity, eating, fever

Answer: (a)   States of mineralocorticoid deficit lead to reduced circulating blood volume as is seen in CHF, hepatic cirrhosis, and nephritic syndrome. Renovascular disorders and coarctation of the aorta, for example, lead to the opposite state of hypertension.

6. Beckwith-Wiedemann syndrome may include the following findings:

   (a) Oligo-amenorrhea, hirsutism, acne, and excessive muscle mass
   (b) Temporal balding, increased libido, and clitoromegaly
   (c) Neonatal macrosomia, macroglossia, and omphalocele

(d) Hyperparathyroidism, pancreatic-duodenal, and pituitary tumors

(e) Islet cell carcinoma of the pancreas, neuroblastoma or hemangiopericytoma

Answer: (c) Neonatal macrosomia, macroglossia and omphalocele comprise the Beckwith-Wiedemann syndrome, which occurs due to an allelic loss of 11q15. The syndrome is associated with adrenocortical tumors along with multiple endocrine neoplasia (MEN) Type 1 (associated with hyperparathyroidism, pancreatic-duodenal and pituitary tumors).

7. Familial pheochromocytomas can occur with or without an association to known syndromes including:

   (a) MEN 1 and the Beckwith-Wiedemann syndrome
   (b) Carney's complex and congenital adrenal hyperplasia
   (c) Li-Fraumeni and McCune-Albright syndromes
   (d) MEN 2, von Hippel-Lindau and neurofibromatosis type 1
   (e) Polycystic ovarian syndrome

Answer: (d) Familial pheochromocytomas can occur with or without the associations described, and are diagnosed at a younger age and tend to have bilateral or multifocal lesions that are usually benign.

8. Pheochromocytomas are:

   (a) Functioning adrenocortical tumors which exhibit elevated levels of several plasma and urinary steroids
   (b) Transitional tumors of sympathetic cell origin which contain elements of both malignant neuroblastoma and benign ganglioneuroma
   (c) Catecholamine-secreting tumors
   (d) Aldosterone-producing adrenocortical carcinomas

(e) Composed of gangliocytes and mature stroma

Answer: (c) Pheochromocytomas are catecholamine-secreting tumors of which 90% originate from the adrenal medulla and 10% arise from extra-adrenal chromaffin tissues (paragangliomas). The tumor is of neuroectodermal origin, and the diagnosis is based on measurements of catecholamine and its metabolic products in plasma or urine.

9. Ganglioneuroblastomas are:

(a) Functioning adrenocortical tumors which exhibit elevated levels of several plasma and urinary steroids
(b) Transitional tumors of sympathetic cell origin which contain elements of both malignant neuroblastoma and benign ganglioneuroma
(c) Catecholamine-secreting tumors
(d) Aldosterone-producing adrenocortical carcinomas
(e) Composed of gangliocytes and mature stroma

Answer: (b) Ganglioneuromas, ganglioneuroblastoma and neuroblastoma are neuroblastic tumors of the sympathetic nervous system. The adrenal glands are the most common site for this tumor and ganglioneuroblastomas are transitional tumors of sympathetic cell origin.

10. Fetal neuroblastoma:

(a) Usually presents with cerebral and, less commonly, renal metastases
(b) Has been discovered as early as 9 weeks
(c) Has a very poor prognosis
(d) May secrete vanillylmandelic acid (VMA) and homovanillic acid (HVA)
(e) Is rarely of adrenal origin

Answer: (d) Since 90% of neuroblastomas secrete VMA and HVA, these urinary catecholamines may be screened to detect the presence of the neoplasm. Fetal neuroblastomas may be discovered as early as 19 weeks and have an excellent prognosis (>90%). These are almost always of adrenal origin and a conservative approach allows involution of these tumors. Newborn screening seems to detect the infant neuroblastomas which often remain occult, regress or mature, and screening has not been shown to decrease the incidence of advanced stage disease in older children nor affect survival.

Surgery of the adrenal

17

CD Anthony Herndon

(Based on chapter written by Stephen Boorjian,
Michael Schwartz, and Dix P Poppas)

1. Advantages to laparoscopic versus open adrenalectomy include all but:

   (a) Improved cosmesis
   (b) Shorter hospital stay
   (c) Cost
   (d) Decreased need for postoperative pain medication
   (e) Quicker return to activity

   Answer: (c) Laparoscopy provides an improvement in cosmesis and postoperative pain management with shorter returns to activity. However, this comes at an increased cost.

2. The fundamental principle for laparoscopic adrenalectomy is:

   (a) Always mobilize the duodenum when approaching the right adrenal gland
   (b) Secure adrenal gland with noncrushing grasper when dissecting gland
   (c) Retroperitoneal access should be attempted prior to transperitoneal dissection
   (d) An attempt should be made to dissect the patient away from the adrenal gland

   Answer: (d) Every attempt should be made *not* to manipulate the adrenal gland during dissection. The surgical dictum "dissect the patient away from the adrenal gland" should be adhered to if at all possible.

3. Advantages in favor of retroperitoneal versus intraperitoneal access include all but:

   (a) Favored in those patients with prior surgery
   (b) Nonadvantageous for those with a history of advanced trauma
   (c) More direct access to the adrenal gland
   (d) May avoid potential intestinal injuries
   (e) Larger working space

   Answer: (e) The main disadvantage to retroperitoneal access is the relatively small working space when compared to intraperitoneal access.

4. In terms of left renal vein anatomic relationships from medial to lateral:

   (a) Lumbar vein, gonadal vein, adrenal vein
   (b) Adrenal vein, lumbar vein, gonadal vein
   (c) Gonadal vein, lumbar vein, adrenal vein
   (d) Adrenal vein, gonadal vein, lumbar vein
   (e) Lumbar vein, adrenal vein, gonadal vein

   Answer: (e) From medial to lateral draining into the renal vein, the lumbar, adrenal and then gonadal veins are encountered.

5. During transperitoneal laparoscopic adrenalectomy which attachments should be taken down last:

   (a) Anterior
   (b) Medial
   (c) Lateral
   (d) Posterior
   (e) Inferior

   Answer: (c) The lateral attachments serve as a retractor that allows dissection of the more medial vascular anatomy.

6. Intraoperative instability may be reduced during an adrenalectomy for a pheochromocytoma by performing all but:

   (a) Aggressive intraoperative hydration
   (b) Minimal adrenal gland manipulation
   (c) Early control of adrenal vein
   (d) Maintaining single agent beta-blockade
   (e) Maintaining single agent calcium channel blockade

Answer: (d)   Patients with a history of pheochromocytoma should be maintained on either calcium-channel blockers or alpha blockers prior to surgery in addition to the above recommendations.

Basic science of the kidney

John C Thomas and John C Pope IV

18

1. Renal agenesis can result from improper signaling between which receptor and ligand:

   (a) Pax-2 and glial cell line-derived neurotrophic factor (GDNF)
   (b) C-ret and GDNF
   (c) Wnt 4 and bone morphogenic protein (BMP) 4
   (d) Transforming growth factor (TGF)-beta and Eya-1

   Answer: (b)   C-ret is a tyrosine kinase receptor located on the tips of the developing ureteral buds that must bind with secreted GDNF from the developing mesenchyme in order to assure normal renal development.

2. Which one of the following is not considered a current potential biomarker for congenital obstructive uropathy:

   (a) Anatomic detail from imaging studies
   (b) Radionuclide scans to determine function
   (c) Molecular markers in the urine
   (d) Microscopic analysis of biopsy specimens

   Answer: (c)   Currently, molecular markers are not used as a biomarker; however, they hold promise in the future to help determine who may need surgical intervention and who can be observed.

3. One difficulty in using animal models to study congenital obstruction in humans is that:

   (a) Rodents and humans have a similar period of nephrogenesis
   (b) Completion of nephrogenesis in animals and humans is different, which makes comparison of postobstructive findings difficult
   (c) An artificially created obstruction is the perfect model to study obstruction which occurs naturally
   (d) Knock-out animals have not helped researchers in defining molecular changes which occur after artificially induced obstruction

   Answer: (b)   Animal models of obstruction are difficult to correlate with obstruction occurring in humans as nephrogenesis is completed at different time points. The closest current model of obstructive uropathy is the neonatal rat, as only 10% of its nephrons are formed at birth, while the rest develop during the first week of life.

4. TGF-beta contributes to fibrosis by:

   (a) Upregulating extracellular matrix proteins and recruiting fibroblasts
   (b) Combining with TGF-alpha to cause cross-linking of collagen
   (c) Suppressing the accumulation of fibronectin, collagen, and proteoglycans
   (d) Downregulating matrix metalloprotein inhibitors
   (e) Inhibiting Smad 3 activation

   Answer: (a)   TGF-beta upregulates extracellular matrix (ECM) proteins and activates the SMAD pathway, including Smad 3, to cause fibrosis. It increases the accumulation of fibronectin, collagen and proteoglycans, and upregulated matrix metalloproteinase (MMP) inhibitors.

5. The RAS is an important contributor to renal fibrosis by which mechanism:

   (a) Increased renin production
   (b) Decreased vascular resistance in the afferent arteriole
   (c) Increasing production of TGF-beta by activating plasminogen activator inhibitor (PAI)-1
   (d) Suppressing apoptosis by decreasing reactive oxygen species (ROS)
   (e) Causes upregulation of MMP inhibitors directly

   Answer: (c) Although important in normal renal development, the RAS can cause or exacerbate fibrosis by increasing human apolipoprotein (apo) AII. AII increases TGF-beta by activating PAI-1, which inhibits the breakdown of plasminogen to plasmin and thereby promotes fibrosis. The RAS promotes apoptosis by increasing ROS.

6. All of the following are potential treatment options except:

   (a) TGF-beta inhibition
   (b) AII receptor blockers
   (c) Nitric oxide activation
   (d) Caspase inhibition
   (e) All of the above

   Answer: (e) All of the listed answers have the potential to limit fibrosis and further apoptosis following obstruction. All of these processes are related to one another so inhibiting one process may have additional benefit by preventing downstream activation of another signaling pathway.

Anomalies of the kidney

Michael Nguyen

(Based on chapter written by Michael Ritchey and Susan John)

1. The kidneys ascend to their final level by the end of which week of fetal life?

   (a) 5th week
   (b) 8th week
   (c) 10th week
   (d) 13th week
   (e) 15th week

   Answer: (b) The kidneys reach their final level by the end of the 8th week of fetal life. Axial rotation medially also occurs during the 7th and 8th week.

2. Failure of induction of the metanephric blastema by the ureteral bud leading to renal agenesis could result from:

   (a) Failure of the ureteral bud or Wolffian duct to develop
   (b) Failure of the ureteral bud to reach the blastema
   (c) Abnormality of the metanephric blastema
   (d) (a) and (c)
   (e) All of the above

   Answer: (e) Abnormalities in any of the interactions between the ureteral bud and metanephric blastema can result in renal agenesis.

3. Which of the following is *false* concerning crossed renal ectopia?

   (a) It is the most common fusion anomaly
   (b) The ectopic kidney crosses the midline to lie on the opposite side from its ureteral insertion

   (c) Crossed renal ectopia with fusion is the most common type of crossed renal ectopia
   (d) There is a slight male predominance
   (e) Crossing from left to right is more common than right to left

   Answer: (a) Crossed renal ectopia is the second most common fusion anomaly behind a horseshoe kidney. The remaining answers are all true regarding crossed renal ectopia.

4. Associated anomalies in children with horseshoe kidneys include:

   (a) Vesicoureteral reflux
   (b) Multicystic dysplasia
   (c) Turner's syndrome
   (d) (a) and (b)
   (e) (a), (b) and (c)

   Answer: (e) All have been found to be associated with a horseshoe kidney. A 7% incidence of horseshoe kidney was noted in patients with Turner's syndrome.

5. Which of the following are *true* regarding anomalies of renal ascent?

   (a) During ascent, the kidney receives its blood supply from the middle sacral artery, iliac artery, and the aorta
   (b) The most common location of an ectopic kidney is in the pelvis opposite the sacrum or below the aortic bifurcation
   (c) Voiding cystourethrogram (VCUG) is not recommended in all children with a diagnosis of pelvic kidney

(d) (a) and (b)

(e) (a), (b) and (c)

Answer: (d) A VCUG is recommended in all children to exclude the diagnosis of vesicoureteral reflux, which is frequently associated with an ectopic kidney.

6. How often is the ipsilateral ureter absent in unilateral renal agenesis?

   (a) 8–15%

   (b) 25–33%

   (c) 50–87%

   (d) 90%

   (e) None of the above

Answer: (c) The ipsilateral ureter is absent in 50–87% of cases of unilateral renal agenesis and only partially developed in others.

7. All of the following are urologic problems found in pelvic kidneys except:

   (a) Renal stones

   (b) Ureteropelvic junction (UPJ) obstruction

   (c) Hydronephrosis

(d) All of the above

(e) None of the above

Answer: (d) The most common urologic problem in pelvic kidneys is a UPJ obstruction due to a high ureteral insertion, or maybe secondary to anomalous vessels that obstruct the UPJ.

8. Which of the following is true regarding a horseshoe kidney?

   (a) The presence of a horseshoe kidney does adversely affect survival

   (b) UPJ obstruction is the second most common cause of hydronephrosis in horseshoe kidneys

   (c) Vesicoureteral reflux is not found in the horseshoe kidney

   (d) Wilms' tumor is the second most common tumor found in horseshoe kidneys

   (e) None of the above

Answer: (d) In a review of National Wilms' Tumor Study patients, there was a sevenfold increased risk of a Wilms' tumor developing in patients with a horseshoe kidney. UPJ obstruction is the most common cause of hydronephrosis in the horseshoe kidney, occurring in 30% of patients.

Fetal and neonatal renal function 21

Paul F Austin

(Based on chapter written by Billy S Arant Jr)

1. In the development of the fetal kidney:

   (a) New glomeruli are formed until 28 weeks gestation
   (b) The human metanephros is formed about 2 weeks after conception
   (c) Each kidney will contain one billion nephrons
   (d) All glomeruli are contained within the cortex
   (e) The essential role of the fetal kidney is to contribute the majority of the amniotic fluid beginning in the first trimester

   Answer: (d)   The other answers are incorrect because:

   • New glomeruli are formed until 34–36 weeks gestation
   • The human metanephros is formed at about the 5th week after conception
   • Each kidney contains approximately one million nephrons
   • The essential role of the fetal kidney is to contribute the majority of the amniotic fluid after the first trimester

2. Which of the following best characterizes the hemodynamics of the fetus?

   (a) Systemic vascular resistance is elevated
   (b) Cardiac output in the fetus and preterm infant is lower than adults
   (c) Vasoactive substances are expressed in low levels in the developing kidney
   (d) Pulmonary and renal circulation vascular resistance is elevated
   (e) Placental circulation ceases after the second trimester

   Answer: (d)   The other answers are incorrect because systemic vascular resistance is kept low in the fetus except in the pulmonary and renal circulations. These regional differences of vascular resistances are in part regulated by vasoactive substances (e.g. angiotensin, prostaglandins and nitric oxide) which are expressed in the developing kidney. Placental circulation continues throughout pregnancy and is interrupted at birth.

3. Renal blood flow in the newborn infant:

   (a) Occurs primarily in the glomeruli residing in the inner cortex
   (b) Is measured by the clearance of inulin
   (c) Increases postnatally as renal vascular resistance decreases
   (d) Is $750\,ml/min/1.73\,m^2$
   (e) Is unaffected by vasoactive factors

   Answer: (c)   Renal blood flow initially is distributed to the glomeruli residing in the outer cortex and becomes evenly distributed to all cortical glomeruli with maturity. This redistribution occurs secondary to vasoactive factors (e.g. angiotensin II) which are also involved in the diminished renal vascular resistance that follows the increase in renal blood flow with birth. Para-aminohippurate (PAH) clearance is the technique for measuring renal blood flow in infants. Renal blood flow in the newborn infant is $290\,ml/min/1.73\,m^2$ and increases with maturity.

4. Which of the following statements is *not* true?

   (a) Glomerular filtration rate (GFR) is low during fetal development until 34 weeks gestation at which time it increases dramatically
   (b) GFR will increase within 1–2 weeks in a 28 week gestational age infant after birth
   (c) The average GFR in the normal adult is 125 ml/min, which is achieved when the average adult body surface area is 1.73 m²
   (d) Developmental changes in GFR occur in every mammalian species
   (e) GFR increases as renal vascular resistance decreases

   Answer: (b)   GFR is low during fetal development until 34 weeks gestation at which time it increases dramatically. This timeline is unaltered in a premature infant. In this example of a 28 week premature infant, GFR will not dramatically increase for 6 more weeks until it reaches 34 weeks corrected gestational age.

5. With respect to GFR:

   (a) After 6 months of age, the absolute value for GFR (ml/min) cannot be corrected for a body surface area of 1.73 m² in a child and compared to adult GFR
   (b) PAH clearance is the technique for measuring GFR in infants
   (c) Nuclear medicine studies are good methods of providing an actual estimate of GFR in infants
   (d) Changes in newborn GFR occur independent of changes in renal vascular resistance
   (e) A serial change in serum creatinine concentration is a clinically useful estimate of GFR in neonates.

   Answer: (e)   The absolute value for GFR (ml/min) can be corrected for a body surface area of 1.73 m² in a child and compared to adult GFR. GFR can be measured directly by a clearance technique that requires a timed urine collection and one or more blood samples using either endogenous creatinine or an exogenous marker such as inulin or iothalimate infused intravenously. There are no normal data published for infants regarding radioisotope techniques to estimate GFR and nuclear medicine studies provide no actual estimate of GFR in infants. The change in GFR which occurs at 34–36 weeks gestation is mediated through changes in renal vascular resistance.

6. With regard to serum creatinine in the infant:

   (a) Serum creatinine concentration will be reduced by 50% during the first week of life in an infant born after 34 weeks gestation
   (b) Premature infants' serum creatinine concentration will be higher than maternal values at birth
   (c) Creatinine clearance is inversely related to GFR
   (d) Normal serum creatinine concentration is approximately 0.7 mg/dl in full-term infants by 1 month of age
   (e) Premature infants will attain a normal serum creatinine concentration comparable to full-term infants by 1 month of age

   Answer: (a)   All newborns, regardless of prematurity, will have maternal values of serum creatinine concentration during the first days of life. Creatinine clearance is directly related to GFR. The normal serum creatinine concentration should be ≤0.4 mg/dl by the end of the first month of life in full-term infants but preterm infants may not reach this level until 3 months of age.

7. Which of the following statements regarding urine volume is *false*:

   (a) Premature infants usually void more frequently and in larger volumes relative to body weight and GFR when compared with full-term infants
   (b) Premature infants have less extracellular fluid to excrete following birth than do full-term infants
   (c) A full-term newborn may not void in the first 12 hours of life
   (d) Initially, the urine is less concentrated in a newborn
   (e) Both premature and full-term infants are capable of concentrating their urine to a specific gravity of >1.020 once extracellular fluid volume has been reduced sufficiently to stimulate the baroreceptor-mediated release of arginine vasopressin from the hypothalamus

Answer: (b) Total body water (TBW) is highest in the preterm infant at 80% body weight. By term, TBW has decreased to 70–75% and continues to fall during the immediate postnatal period to 60–65% during the latter part of the first year of life. The extracellular fluid compartment comprises the bulk of the TBW and parallels this decrease by percent body weight with maturity: 60% body weight in the premature infant; 45% in the term infant; and 30% in the adolescent.

8. Markers for the end of the postnatal diuresis in a normal infant, regardless of maturity, are:

   (a) A reduction in the frequency and volume of urine excreted
   (b) An increase in urinary osmolarity
   (c) A stabilization of the infant's body weight
   (d) (a) and (c)
   (e) All of the above

Answer: (e) Each statement is a marker for the end of postnatal diuresis.

9. Which of the following statements regarding tubular handling of sodium is *false*:

   (a) Classic teaching previously touted that premature infants could not conserve sodium and full-term infants could not excrete sodium
   (b) Renal handling of sodium is reflective of changes in effective arterial blood volume
   (c) The status of effective arterial blood volume overrides any signaling from body fluid osmolarity
   (d) The fractional excretion of sodium (FENa) is <1% in the setting of diuretics, obstruction or fluid overload
   (e) An increase in the effective arterial blood volume results in the renal excretion of sodium and water in the mature kidney

Answer: (d) FENa will increase >1% with an increase in effective arterial blood volume, by tubular injury as with diuretics, obstruction or renal disease, or by any maneuver which increases the fractional excretion of water such as fluid overload.

10. Which of the following statements regarding acid–base balance is *false*:

   (a) Unless demand becomes overwhelming, the neonatal kidney is capable of reabsorbing bicarbonate filtered by the glomerulus and secreting hydrogen ions
   (b) An increased effective arterial blood volume results in reabsorption of all substances presented to the distal tubule
   (c) Most of the acidemia measured in premature infants can be accounted for by respiratory acidosis
   (d) Most so-called renal tubular acidosis in infants is a complication of diarrheal disease with the intestinal loss of bicarbonate

(e) Distal tubular injury from obstruction or infection impairs the ability of that part of the nephron to secrete hydrogen ions and potassium, resulting in a metabolic acidosis and hyperkalemia.

Answer: (b)   An increased effective arterial blood volume results in reabsorption of all substances presented to the *proximal* tubule – not just sodium and chloride, but also bicarbonate.

Cystic kidney disease

22

Larry A Greenbaum

1. Which of the following cell structures appears to be involved in cyst formation in a variety of inherited cystic kidney diseases?

   (a) Mitochondria
   (b) Primary cilium
   (c) Lysosomes
   (d) Ribosomes
   (e) Nuclear pores

   Answer: (b) In a variety of cystic kidney diseases – including autosomal dominant polycystic kidney disease, autosomal recessive polycystic kidney disease, and nephronophthisis – there are mutations in genes encoding proteins which are components of or associated with the primary cilium of renal tubular cells.

2. You palpate an enlarged liver in a 6-year-old child with autosomal recessive polycystic kidney disease. What is the likely etiology?

   (a) Intrahepatic aneurysm
   (b) Autoimmune hepatitis
   (c) Liver cysts
   (d) Liver displacement due to enlarged kidneys
   (e) Hepatic fibrosis

   Answer: (e) Hepatic fibrosis occurs in patients with autosomal recessive kidney disease. Clinical consequences of hepatic fibrosis include cholangitis and manifestations of portal hypertension such as esophageal varices and splenomegaly.

3. Which of the following diseases is likely to present clinically during the first year of life?

   (a) Nephronophthisis
   (b) Medullary cystic kidney disease

   (c) Autosomal recessive cystic kidney disease
   (d) Autosomal dominant cystic kidney disease
   (e) Medullary sponge kidney

   Answer: (c) The majority of patients with autosomal recessive polycystic kidney disease present during the first year of life, with a significant percentage being diagnosed during the neonatal period. The other entities are typically diagnosed later in childhood or in adults.

4. A 14-year-old child is seen in your office because of gross hematuria, which occurred during football practice. Among cystic kidney diseases, which of the following is the most likely diagnosis?

   (a) Nephronophthisis
   (b) Medullary cystic kidney disease
   (c) Autosomal recessive cystic kidney disease
   (d) Autosomal dominant cystic kidney disease
   (e) Multicystic dysplastic kidney

   Answer: (d) Hematuria occurs in patients with autosomal dominant polycystic kidney disease and the hematuria may be associated with physical activity. Gross hematuria is rarely reported in the other entities.

5. You are seeing a patient with autosomal dominant polycystic kidney disease. Which of the following is *not* a possible extrarenal manifestation?

   (a) Ruptured intracranial aneurysm
   (b) Hepatic cysts
   (c) Tapetoretinal degeneration

(d) Inguinal hernia

(e) Mitral valve prolapse

Answer: (c)   Mitral valve prolapse and inguinal hernias are more common in children with autosomal dominant polycystic kidney disease (ADPKD). Ruptured intracranial aneurysms and hepatic cysts are rare in children with ADPKD, but occur in adults. Tapetoretinal degeneration does not occur in ADPKD.

6. You are seeing a 9-year-old boy due to primary nocturnal enuresis. By history, he has polydipsia and polyuria. He also craves salty foods. What cystic kidney disease do you need to consider in your differential diagnosis?

(a) Nephronophthisis

(b) Medullary sponge kidney

(c) Autosomal recessive cystic kidney disease

(d) Autosomal dominant cystic kidney disease

(e) Multicystic dysplastic kidney

Answer: (a)   High urine output and salt wasting are common in nephronophthisis. This leads to polydipsia, and may cause enuresis and salt craving. The high urine output persists even when patients develop renal failure.

7. What is the typical outcome in a child with bilateral multicystic dysplastic kidney disease?

(a) Senior Loken syndrome

(b) Potter syndrome

(c) Pomeranz syndrome

(d) Fanconi syndrome

(e) Ask-Upmark syndrome

Answer: (b)   Children with bilateral multicystic dysplastic kidneys die at birth due to Potter syndrome, which is caused by severe oligohydramnios. Manifestations of Potter syndrome include facial features (hypertelorism, low-set ears, receding chin, and flattening

of the nose), limb deformities, and pulmonary hypoplasia that is incompatible with life.

8. You are seeing a neonate with a unilateral multicystic dysplastic kidney (MCDK) that was detected on prenatal ultrasound. The diagnosis was confirmed by a postnatal renal ultrasound. You should tell the parents:

(a) The child requires immediate nephrectomy of the MCDK to prevent malignant transformation

(b) The child should have a nephrectomy of the MCDK at about 1 year of age

(c) The child requires regular renal ultrasound follow-up

(d) No further follow-up is indicated since the contralateral kidney is normal

(e) The child may develop cysts in the contralateral kidney

Answer: (c)   MCDK are typically asymptomatic and the majority completely involute and disappear during the first 6 years of life. Hence, routine nephrectomy is no longer recommended. Ultrasound follow-up is currently recommended due to an extremely low risk of malignant transformation.

9. You are seeing a 1-year-old child with a unilateral MCDK. The child is otherwise healthy. The parents are now considering having a second child and they want to know the risk of a MCDK in subsequent children. What is the inheritance of MCDK?

(a) Autosomal recessive

(b) Autosomal dominant

(c) X-linked recessive

(d) Genetic imprinting

(e) None of the above

Answer: (e)   Most cases of MCDK are sporadic, without a genetic etiology. There are a few families described with putative autosomal dominant inheritance and MCDK is increased in certain genetic syndromes.

10. Which of the following diseases can be associated with cystic kidney disease?

    (a) Tuberous sclerosis
    (b) Neurofibromatosis
    (c) Cystic fibrosis
    (d) Gordon syndrome
    (e) Sickle-cell disease

Answer: (a) Tuberous sclerosis, one of the neurocutaneous syndromes, has significant renal manifestations. Angiomyolipomas are the most frequent complication, and they may cause bleeding and renal insufficiency in late childhood and adulthood. Cysts are less common and are often due to a chromosomal deletion which affects two adjacent genes: one of the tuberous sclerosis genes and one of the autosomal dominant polycystic kidney disease genes.

Acute renal failure

23

Lawrence Copelovitch, Bernard S Kaplan, and Kevin EC Meyers

1. Acute renal failure (ARF) may be associated with which of the following?

   (a) Anuria
   (b) Oliguria
   (c) Polyuria
   (d) Normal urine output
   (e) All of the above

   Answer: (e) Acute renal failure, the sudden decrease in normal kidney function compromises normal renal regulation of fluid, electrolyte, and acid–base homeostasis. ARF is a reduction in glomerular filtration rate (GFR), which results in an increase in the creatinine and blood urea nitrogen, and may be characterized with anuria, oliguria, polyuria or normal urine output.

2. Which of the following is usually associated with nonoliguric ARF?

   (a) The maintenance phase of ischemic-induced acute tubular necrosis (ATN)
   (b) Acute interstitial nephritis
   (c) Dehydration
   (d) Acute glomurelonephritis
   (e) Cardiac tamponade

   Answer: (b) Children with acute interstitial nephritis or nephrotoxicity from medications are more likely to have normal or increased urine output ARF. The maintenance phase of ischemia-induced ATN, acute glomerulo-nephritis, and dehydration are characterized by oliguria.

3. Which of the following is associated with a high likelihood of recovery in ARF?

   (a) Oliguria
   (b) Multiple organ dysfunction
   (c) Requirement for dialysis
   (d) Polyuria
   (e) Prolonged renal insult

   Answer: (d) Recovery from ARF is predicated on the amount of urine output and the underlying cause. Patients with nonoliguric or high-output ARF have lower complication rates and higher survival rates than those with anuria or oliguric ARF.

4. Which of the following is *not* an endogenous toxin which can cause ATN?

   (a) Myoglobin
   (b) Hemoglobin
   (c) Methemoglobin
   (d) Uric acid

   Answer: (c) Myoglobin or hemoglobin-induced ARF is more likely to develop in the presence of dehydration, metabolic acidosis or multiple organ failure as the pigment may precipitate in the tubules and cause tubular injury. Uric acid may similarly precipitate in tubules while methemoglobinemia does not cause ATN.

5. Which of the following is *not* a common metabolic complication of ARF?

   (a) Hypernatremia
   (b) Hypocalcemia
   (c) Hyperkalemia
   (d) Hyperphosphatemia
   (e) Metabolic acidosis

   Answer: (a)   Serum electrolytes are carefully monitored in a patient with ARF as they are important guides to predicting morbidity and mortality. Hyponatremia may occur due to fluid overload, but hypernatremia is not commonly seen with ARF. The remainder of the choices above are also common metabolic complications.

6. Which of the following is an indication for initiating dialysis?

   (a) Volume overload unresponsive to conservative management
   (b) Hyperkalemia unresponsive to medical therapy
   (c) Uremia
   (d) Prolonged malnutrition
   (e) All of the above

   Answer: (e)   All of the above, as well as the patient's overall condition, must be evaluated before dialysis is considered.

7. Which is not a principle in the management of ARF?

   (a) Maintain renal perfusion
   (b) Administer large volumes of isotonic crystalloid regardless of volume status
   (c) Avoid nephrotoxic agents
   (d) Maintain electrolyte balance
   (e) Provide nutritional support

   Answer: (b)   Renal hypoperfusion is a predisposing factor to developing ARF, so establishing a fluid balance is critical in management. The volume of resuscitation depends very much on the fluid status of the patient and whether the ARF is oliguric, anuric or polyuric.

8. Which of the following is incorrect with regards to urine studies?

   (a) A high urine specific gravity suggests prerenal ARF
   (b) Red blood cell casts strongly suggest a glomerular lesion
   (c) Significant proteinuria ($>3+$) is highly suggestive of ATN
   (d) A low fractional excretion of sodium ($<1\%$) suggests prerenal ARF
   (e) A positive dipstick for blood with no red blood cells on microscopic examination is suggestive of myoglobinuria

   Answer: (c)   A dipstick test revealing significant proteinuria indicates intrinsic ARF with glomerular damage and not ATN. Prerenal ARF, ATN, and postrenal ARF are indicated by less proteinuria.

9. Which of the following agents has been associated with toxin-mediated ATN?

   (a) Amphotericin
   (b) Aminoglycosides
   (c) Acyclovir
   (d) Ethylene glycol
   (e) All of the above

   Answer: (e)   Renal injury from toxins usually presents with a decrease in urine concentrating capacity, and is usually transient, mild and nonoliguric. Risk factors include extremes of age, hypovolemia, and preexisting renal insufficiency.

10. Pyelonephritis falls into which category of intrinsic renal disease?

    (a) Interstitial
    (b) Glomerular
    (c) Vascular

(d) Tubular
(e) None of the above

Answer: (a)   Pyelonephritis, systemic diseases, tumor infiltrates or genetic conditions most result in interstitial injury. Fever, rash, arthralgias and flank pain are typical symptoms. Urine output is usually increased or normal and interstitial injury is the most frequent cause of nonoliguric ARF.

Renal transplantation

24

Nafisa Dharamsi, Curtis Sheldon, and Jens Gobel

1. If a short renal vein is encountered during a renal transplant then:

   (a) It can be extended by using adjacent cavil flaps
   (b) A small patch of cava or aorta can be used to provide the extension
   (c) The recipient venous tree is mobilized extensively
   (d) Vascular reconstruction is completed with techniques of dividing and spatulating the renal vein

   Answer: (c) In most cases, if a short renal vein is encountered, additional length can be gained by mobilizing the recipient venous tree. If this is not sufficient to create a tension-free anastomosis, the renal vein can be extended by tubularizing adjacent caval flaps.

2. Ureteral stents are utilized in transplants for all the following reasons except:

   (a) To prevent ureteral obstruction from anastomotic edema
   (b) To decrease potential risk of extravasation
   (c) To maximize ureteral vascularity
   (d) To prevent clot colic postoperatively
   (e) To increase intrarenal reflux postoperatively

   Answer: (e) All are true and stents do increase reflux into the kidney, however, they are not utilized for this purpose during renal transplantation. The stents are utilized to prevent ureteral obstruction from anastomotic edema, to decrease extravasation from the anastomosis, to stabilize the ureter thereby maximizing ureteral vascularity and to prevent clot colic.

3. Advantages of the extravesical approach to ureteral reimplant include all the following except:

   (a) Shortening operating room time
   (b) Low incidence of anastomotic obstruction
   (c) Reduction in postoperative hematuria
   (d) Reduction in urinary extravasation
   (e) Decreased risk of vesicoureteral reflux

   Answer: (d) Options for the ureterovesical reimplantation include transvesically or extravesically. Advantages of the extravesical approach include all of the above except for reducing urinary extravasation post-operatively.

4. The best solution for preservation of all abdominal organs is:

   (a) EuroCollins
   (b) Ringer's lactated solution with heparin
   (c) Sach's solution
   (d) Collins 2
   (e) University of Wisconsin (UW) solution

   Answer: (e) University of Wisconsin solution favors graft function and survival over EuroCollins.

5. The standard method of reconstructing the ureter during the renal transplant is:

   (a) Ureteropyelostomy
   (b) Ureteroureterostomy

(c) Cutaneous ureterostomy

(d) Ureteroneocystotomy

(e) Transureteroureterostomy

Answer: (d) The ureter is most commonly reimplanted into the bladder – ureteroneocystotomy – using a transvesical or extravesical approach. A less frequently used option is (b) and, rarely, (a), (c) and (e).

6. Etiology of urolithiasis posttransplantation includes all the following except:

(a) Retained suture material

(b) High citrate and low phosphate excretion in the urine

(c) Decreased urine output

(d) Alkaline urine

(e) Increased frequency of urinary tract infections and urine stasis

Answer: (b) Urolithiasis is seen after 5% of pediatric renal transplants. The etiology of the stones is multifactorial; however, retained suture material, decreased urine output, alkaline urine, and increased frequency of urinary tract infections would all facilitate stone formation. High citrate is protective against urolithiasis.

7. All of the following are indications for pretransplant nephrectomy except:

(a) Renal tumor

(b) Hypertension controlled with one agent

(c) Severe hydronephrosis

(d) Recurrent renal infection

(e) Stones not managed with minimally invasive procedures

Answer: (b) All of the above are indications for pretransplant nephrectomy except hypertension, which can be controlled with one agent. If, however, the hypertension cannot be controlled easily with one agent, a nephrectomy should be considered.

8. Common causes of end-stage renal disease (ESRD) in children are all of the below except:

(a) Focal segmental glomerulosclerosis

(b) Obstructive uropathy, e.g. from posterior urethral valves

(c) Renal dysplasia

(d) Diabetic nephropathy

(e) Reflux nephropathy

Answer: (d) The common causes of ESRD in children are different from adults where diabetes and hypertension play a large role. The common causes in children are the congenital obstructive and dysplastic conditions.

9. Kidney transplantation is contraindicated in the presence of:

(a) Malignancy

(b) Chronic infection, e.g. tuberculosis

(c) Significant noncompliance

(d) Ongoing substance abuse

(e) All of the above

Answer: (e) Contraindications are potentially modifiable with "safe" periods after curative treatment for malignancy and chronic infections are available. Some centers offer kidney transplantation to certain patients infected with human immunodeficiency virus: noncompliance and substance abuse can be overcome in some instances. However, these all need to be addressed carefully.

10. Commonly used immunosuppressants in pediatric kidney transplantation include:

(a) A calcineurin inhibitor

(b) A corticosteroid

(c) Rapamycin

(d) Mycophenolate mofetil

(e) All of the above

Answer: (e) Given the relatively small number of pediatric kidney transplants and the increasing number of drugs available, most evidence for immunosuppressive regimens is derived from adult studies. A typical protocol to be used initially in pediatric kidney transplantation currently consists of triple therapy with a calcineurin inhibitor (CI) and steroids, possibly paired with a course of induction with a nondepleting anti-T cell antibody. However, these are constantly changing and adjusted to individualized treatment based on the recipient's estimated risk for acute rejection balanced against side-effects. New treatment protocols are attempting to avoid steroids completely and to reduce the use of CIs.

11. Complications seen with increased frequency when transplanting laparoscopically obtained adult kidneys specifically into small children are:

(a) Delayed graft function and rejection
(b) Infection and malignancy
(c) Wound dehiscence and respiratory compromise
(d) Cardiovascular compromise and decreased end-organ perfusion
(e) Ureteral anastomotic insufficiency

Answer: (a) Small children, less than the age of 5, have repeatedly been shown to have inferior outcomes in terms of delayed graft function and early rejection following a laparoscopic nephrectomy.[1] Graft survival and rejection rates in older children appear not to differ on the method of harvest.

12. Enhanced immunosuppression should be considered in the setting of:

(a) Poor human leukocyte antigen (HLA) matching
(b) Recipient presensitization
(c) Delayed graft function/acute tubular necrosis
(d) African-American recipient race
(e) All of the above

Answer: (e) Least powerful antirejection prophylaxis is required by first-time Caucasian recipients of a live donor kidney who have no evidence of presensitization. Enhanced immunosuppresion is required when: the recipient is of a repeat transplant, especially one from a deceased donor; the recipient has evidence of presensitization; the recipient is African-American.

13. In the immediate posttransplant period, the intravascular volume of pediatric recipients of functioning kidneys from adult donors needs to be:

(a) Aggressively restricted to prevent pulmonary edema, hypertension and congestive heart failure
(b) Restricted to balance the avid tendency of freshly transplanted kidneys to concentrate the urine
(c) Generous to provide good perfusion of the new allograft
(d) Generous to compensate for the typically limited ability of freshly transplanted kidneys to concentrate the urine
(e) (c) and (d)

Answer: (e) The relatively large adult donor kidney in a pediatric recipient requires excellent perfusion – recommendations include a central venous pressure (CVP) between 12 and $16\,cmH_2O$ to provide adequate renal turgor. The generous requirements to maintain a central venous pressure sufficient for good blood flow to the transplant persist during and after the surgery may continue long term, with even night-time or bolus supplementations being required.

14. Not included in the differential diagnosis of early allograft dysfunction is:

(a) Acute rejection
(b) Acute CI toxicity
(c) Vascular thrombosis

(d) Chronic allograft nephropathy (CAN)

(e) Urinary tract obstruction

Answer: (d)   Early allograft dysfunction is triggered by all of the above except CAN, which is a long-term complication affecting kidney transplant recipients. Other long-term complications include the high incidence of cardiovascular (CV) disease and malignancies compared to the general population.

15. The age group of pediatric kidney transplant recipients at highest risk for adverse outcomes, in part because of noncompliance, is:

(a) Infants

(b) Preschoolers

(c) Preteens

(d) Teenagers

(e) Young adults

Answer: (d)   Transplantation is a complex therapy that requires adherence and close follow-up. It has been documented that only 50% of patients will adhere to a long-term medical regimen and studies have shown that most noncompliant patients are teenagers. These children are more likely to lose their grafts and have demonstrably poorer renal function. Noncomplaint teenagers are more often girls than boys and frequently the cause for the noncompliance is due to the side-effect profile of the immunosuppressant.

16. Challenges ahead in the management of pediatric kidney transplant recipients are:

(a) Chronic allograft nephropathy

(b) Accelerated CV disease

(c) Skeletal problems, e.g. suboptimal growth

(d) Malignancies such as posttransplant lymphoproliferative disease and infections as indicators of overimmunosuppression

(e) All of the above

Answer: (e)

Reference

1. Troppman C, McBride MA, Baker TJ, Perez RV. Laparoscopic live donor nephrectomy: a risk factor for delayed function and rejection in pediatric kidney recipients? A UNOS analysis. Am J Transplant 2005; 5: 175–82.

Renal calculus disease

25

Parmod Reddy and Eugene Minevich

1. The prevalence of hypercalciuria is greater in pediatric patients with vesicoureteral reflux (VUR) than in the general population. True or False?

   Answer: True The high prevalence of hypercalciuria found in the parents, and the high prevalence of urolithiasis in other relatives of children with VUR, points to a genetic origin of the hypercalciuria. Data suggest that the inheritance of hypercalciuria in patients with VUR is autosomal dominant as it has been described for idiopathic hypercalciuria, although with a higher probability to be inherited from the mother. This may be due to a mechanism known as genetic imprinting, which has been observed in many autosomal dominant transmitted diseases in which an autosomal gene has a different behavior depending on the parent from whom it has been inherited.[1,2]

2. Which of the following conditions are inherited in an autosomal recessive manner?

   (a) Cystinuria
   (b) Renal tubular acidosis
   (c) Primary hyperoxaluria
   (d) (a) and (b)
   (e) (a) and (c)

   Answer: (e) Cystinuria and primary hyperoxaluria are inherited as autosomal recessive disorders, whereas renal tubular acidosis and the syndrome of idiopathic calcium oxalate urolithiasis are inherited as autosomal dominant conditions.

Cystinuria is an autosomal recessive defect in reabsorptive transport of cystine and the dibasic amino acids ornithine, arginine, and lysine from the luminal fluid of the renal proximal tubule and small intestine. The clinical manifestation of cystinuria is cystine urolithiasis, which often recurs throughout a patient's lifetime. Surgical intervention is often necessary to treat the calculi.

Primary hyperoxaluria is a very rare but serious disorder caused by a congenital defect, resulting in very high levels ($>200\,mg/d$) of endogenous oxalate production. Renal failure develops in 80% of these patients by the third decade. Normal dialysis for uremia cannot remove enough serum oxalate to protect the kidneys and other organs from widespread calcium oxalate deposition (i.e. oxalosis) and calcium oxalate stone production. Type I hyperoxaluria is the more common variety. It occurs in 1 per 120,000 live births and is transmitted as an autosomal recessive trait, caused by a deficiency of the peroxisomal liver-specific alanine:glyoxylate aminotransferase gene (AGT). The median age for presentation of initial symptoms related to hyperoxaluria is 5 years. Oxalate deposition occurs in multiple organs (e.g. bones, joints, eyes, heart). In particular, bone tends to be the major repository of excess oxalate in patients with primary hyperoxaluria. It is recommended that all pediatric patients who have stones should be screened for hyperoxaluria. The discovery of the condition in a child permits the siblings to be screened for the disease and preemptive treatment. Liver transplantation prior to the development of overt renal failure may preserve the individual's native renal function, thus avoiding renal transplantation. Renal transplantation alone is insufficient because the liver defect causing the hyperoxaluria is not corrected. Type II hyperoxaluria is due to a deficiency of D-glyceric dehydrogenase and this condition is less common than type I. End-stage renal disease is slightly less common in patients with type II primary hyperoxaluria.[3,4]

3. The most common cause of hypocitriuria in children is:

(a) Renal tubular acidosis
(b) Hypokalemia
(c) Urinary tract infection (UTI)
(d) (a) and (b)
(e) (b) and (c)

Answer: (a) Hypocitriuria is defined as urinary citrate excretion of <250 mg in 24 hours. Urinary citrate forms a soluble complex with calcium which inhibits the formation and propagation of crystals. It is a common correctable cause of recurrent calcium stones. Females excrete more citrate and have lower incidence of stone formation than age-matched males. Urinary citrate is mainly derived endogenously through the tricarboxylic acid cycle and is excreted by renal tubular cells. Intracellular acidosis, acidic diets (diets rich in animal proteins), and hypokalemia decrease urinary citrate excretion. Fruits such as oranges and grapefruits are the main exogenous sources of urinary citrate. Hypocitraturia in type I renal tubular acidosis is thought to be due to a defect in distal tubule function.

4. The enzyme deficiency that results in primary hyperoxaluria is:

(a) Hypoxanthine-guanine phosphoribosyl transferase (HPRT)
(b) 1,8 Dihydroxyadenyl transferase
(c) Xanthine dehydrogenase
(d) Glyceraldehyde-3-phosphate dehydrogenase (GAPDH)
(e) Hepatic peroxisomal alanine-glyoxylate

Answer: (e) The enzyme deficiency in primary hyperoxaluria is hepatic peroxisomal alanine-glyoxylate, therefore the only treatment for these patients is a liver transplant.[4]

5. The enzyme deficiency that results in Lesch-Nyhan syndrome is:

(a) GAPDH
(b) 1,8 Dihydroxyadenyl transferase
(c) HPRT
(d) Xanthine dehydrogenase
(e) Hepatic peroxisomal alanine-glyoxylate

Answer: (c) Lesch-Nyhan syndrome is a condition that results in hyperuricosuria and is due to a deficiency of the enzyme HPRT. Lesch-Nyhan syndrome is inherited as an X-linked disease, therefore the disease is seen mainly in males. It is characterized by increased blood and urine uric acid levels. The features of the Lesch-Nyhan syndrome are mental retardation, spastic cerebral palsy, choreoathetosis, uric acid urinary stones, and self-destructive biting of fingers and lips. The excess uric acid levels cause children to develop gout-like swelling in some of their joints. Uric acid urolithiasis and renal dysfunction develop because of the excess uric acid levels.[5]

6. Which of the following is/are naturally occurring inorganic inhibitors in urine that affect the Ksp (solubility product) of lithogenic ions?

(a) Magnesium
(b) Sodium
(c) Calcium
(d) Nephrocalcin
(e) (a) and (d)

Answer: (a) The supersaturation theory is based on the binding of salts, which occurs after a certain concentration is obtained.

A compound's thermodynamic solubility product (Ksp) defines the saturation of a compound in a solution. The Ksp of a compound is equal to the product of a pure chemical in equilibrium between a solid and solvent in solution. If a compound's concentration exceeds the Ksp, it precipitates. Temperature, pH, and the presence of inhibitors or promoters in the solution also affect the compound's solubility. Magnesium is an inorganic inhibitor that is found in urine and serves as an inhibitor of lithogenesis. While nephrocalcin is also an inhibitor found in urine it is an organic compound. Sodium and calcium promote lithogenesis.[6]

7. Where does lithogenesis (urinary crystal formation) begin?

(a) Glomerulus
(b) Efferent duct
(c) Ascending loop of Henle
(d) Papillary duct
(e) Renal pelvis

Answer: (d) The papillary duct is the site of initial crystal formation and retention, which subsequently results in stone formation.

8. Important factors that are relevant in the medical history of a child with urolithiasis are:

(a) Recurrent skeletal fractures
(b) Prematurity
(c) Nutritional habits
(d) Failure to thrive
(e) All of the above

Answer: (e) While obtaining a history in a child with urolithiasis one should be sure to ask about the following:

- History of prematurity, especially the use of furosemide or calcium supplements during the new-born period
- History of recurrent skeletal fractures – ?hyperparathyroidism

- History of concurrent diseases such as cystic fibrosis, neoplasms, etc.
- Nutritional habits – ketogenic diet

Failure to thrive might indicate underlying gastrointestinal (GI) malabsortive conditions, renal tubular acidosis.

9. The single most important predisposing metabolic factor in pediatric urolithiasis is:

(a) Hyperuricosuria
(b) Hyperoxaluria
(c) Hypovolemia
(d) Hypercalciuria
(e) Hypocitriuria

Answer: (d) Hypercalciuria is the single most important risk factor in the development of pediatric urolithiasis. Hypercalciuira occurs in 53–81% of all children with calcium stones.[7]

10. What is the underlying defect in the type of renal tubular acidosis which is associated with stone formation?

(a) Failure of bicarbonate reabsorption in the proximal tubule
(b) Chronic renal parenchymal damage
(c) Hyperchloremic metabolic acidosis
(d) Inability of the distal nephron to maintain a hydrogen ion gradient between the tubular fluid and the blood
(e) Bicarbonate wasting

Answer: (d) Renal tubular acidosis is a term applied to several conditions in which metabolic acidosis is caused by specific defects in renal tubular hydrogen ion secretion. Three types of renal tubular acidosis are generally recognized based on the nature of the tubular defect. Nephrolithiasis occurs only in type I renal tubular acidosis, a condition marked by an abnormality in the generation and maintenance of a hydrogen ion gradient by the distal tubule. Type I renal tubular acidosis is a heterogeneous disorder which may be hereditary, idiopathic or secondary to a variety of conditions.[8]

References

1. García-Nieto V, Siverio B, Monge M, Toledo C, Molini N. Urinary calcium excretion in children with vesicoureteral reflux. Nephrol Dial Transplant 2003; 18: 507–11.
2. Guizar J, Kornhauser C, Malacara J, Sanchez G, Zamora J. Renal tubular acidosis in children with vesicoureteral reflux. J Urol 1996; 156: 193–5.
3. Chow GK, Streem SB. Contemporary urological intervention for cystinuric patients: immediate and long-term impact and implications. J Urol 1998; 160: 341–4; discussion 344–5.
4. Cochat P, Basmaison O. Current approaches to the management of primary hyperoxaluria. Arch Dis Child 2000; 82: 470–3.
5. Nyhan WL, Wong DF. New approaches to understanding Lesch-Nyhan disease. N Engl J Med 1996; 334: 1602–4.
6. Schrier RW. Diseases of the Kidney and Urinary Tract. Philadelphia: Lippincott Williams & Wilkins, 2006.
7. Rudolph AM, Kamei RK, Overby KJ. Rudolph's Fundamentals of Pediatrics. New York: McGraw-Hill, 2002.
8. Rodríguez-Soriano J. New insights into the pathogenesis of renal tubular acidosis – from functional to molecular studies. Pediatr Nephrol 2000; 14: 1121–36.

Endourology for stone disease 26

Steven Lukasewycz and Aseem R Shukla

(Based on chapter by Aseem R Shukla and Michael Erhard)

1. What percentage of pediatric patients diagnosed with urolithiasis complain of flank pain at initial evaluation?

   (a) 10%
   (b) 20%
   (c) 40%
   (d) 50%
   (e) 80%

   Answer: (d)   Only 50% of pediatric patients diagnosed with urolithaisis complain of flank pain. The other common presentations include gross or microscopic hematuria, incidental findings, and urinary tract infections.

2. In the evaluation for pediatric urolithiasis ultrasound has:

   (a) Equivalent sensitivity when compared to computerized tomography (CT)
   (b) No role in the contemporary evaluation of renal stones
   (c) Increased sensitivity when compared to CT
   (d) Decreased sensitivity when compared to CT
   (e) None of the above

   Answer: (d)   Although ultrasound is often the first choice of imaging modality in the pediatric population – and does demonstrate large renal calculi or presence of hydronephrosis – it has very low sensitivity for detecting urolithiasis, especially for stones located in the ureter. While radiation exposure is certainly a concern in the pediatric population, a noncontrast helical CT is the "gold standard" for detecting urolithiasis.

3. One hour after undergoing extracorporeal shock-wave lithotripsy (SWL) for a 1 cm right renal pelvic stone a 13-year-old female patient complains of excruciating right-sided flank pain. On examination, vital signs are stable and examination reveals no ecchymosis. KUB shows stone fragments in the renal pelvis but no evidence of ureteral calculi. The next step is:

   (a) Administration of morphine to decrease expected postoperative pain
   (b) Administration of ketorolac to decrease expected postoperative pain
   (c) Ureteroscopy to evaluate and remove stone fragments
   (d) Renal ultrasound to evaluate for perinephric hematoma
   (e) Transfusion

   Answer: (d)   Though uncommon, clinically significant subcapsular hematoma can occur after SWL. Often, these patients present with extreme flank pain though they are clinically otherwise stable. Evaluation should include ultrasound or CT scan to evaluate for this condition, but only conservative management and observation are typically required.

4. Hydrophilic-coated guidewires are best used for/as:

   (a) Initial cannulization of the ureteral orifice to minimize trauma

(b) A safety wire because the hydrophilic coating allows other instruments to pass with minimal resistance

(c) Getting access past an impacted ureteral stone or narrow stricture

(d) Percutaneous tract dilation

(e) All of the above

Answer: (c) Hydrophilic-coated guidewires are primarily used for negotiating tortuous and narrowed ureters, and for gaining wire access past an impacted stone. These wires are often extremely slippery and therefore are not used for routine access of the ureteral orifice or as a safety wire as they can become easily dislodged. Extra-stiff guidewires are chosen for percutaneous tract dilation.

5. Which of the following statements are *true* regarding intracorporeal lithotripsy?

(a) Ultrasonic lithotripsy can be effectively performed through a flexible nephroscope

(b) Shortcomings of ballistic lithotripsy include loss of power with instrument deflection and retrograde stone migration

(c) Electrohydraulic lithotripsy (EHL) facilitates stone fragmentation by creation of a cavitation bubble with maximal energy 5 mm from the probe tip

(d) Due to the differential absorption of the Ho:YAG laser, damage to urothelium or the endoscope is not a significant concern

Answer: (b) Ultrasonic lithotripsy probes lose power with deflection and therefore are not effectively used through flexible scopes. EHL does produce stone fragmentation through creation of a cavitation bubble and maximal power is approximately 1 mm from the probe tip. Though very effective for stone fragmentation, Ho:YAG can cause significant damage to both urothelium and equipment. Only (b) is true in that ballistic (pneumatic) lithotripsy probes may lose

power with instrument deflection and retrograde stone migration are shortcomings of ballistic lithotripsy.

6. All of the following methods are commonly used to access a narrow ureteral orifice for ureteroscopy *except*:

(a) Soft graduated ureteral dilator

(b) Pre-stenting the ureter for passive dilation

(c) Balloon dilation of ureteral orifice

(d) Incision of the ureteral orifice with a Ho:YAG laser

Answer: (d) Though ureteroscopy can be effectively performed in the pediatric population, ureteral dilation is necessary in approximately 30% of children undergoing this procedure. Options for dilation include use of a graduated single-shaft dilator, balloon dilation or temporary placement of a ureteral stent. An incision with laser may be considered for a ureteral stricture, but this is unusual for standard ureteroscopy.

7. Ureteroscopic stone extraction should be considered first-line treatment for ureteral stones in the pediatric population. True or False?

Answer: True According to the American Urological Association (AUA) treatment guidelines ureteroscopic stone extraction is safe and effective in the pediatric population, and should be considered first-line treatment.

8. Factors that are likely to decrease stone-free rates for ESWL monotherapy include which of the following?

(a) Presence of an ectopic kidney

(b) Presence of cysteine stones

(c) Stone within a narrow-neck calyceal diverticulum

(d) Stones within a narrowed lower pole infundibulum

(e) All of the above

Answer: (e)   ESWL can be quite efficacious in the pediatric population with stone-free rates quoted at >80%. However, several factors decrease the effectiveness of ESWL therapy including presence of an ectopic or horseshoe kidney, presence of "hard stones" such as cysteine or brushite stones, stones within calyceal diverticula, and stones within elongated narrowed lower pole infundibula.

9. Which factors have been shown to decrease transfusion rates in the pediatric population?

    (a) Use of an access tract <22F
    (b) Use of an access tract <12F
    (c) Use of a single as opposed to multiple access tracts
    (d) None of the above
    (e) (a) and (c)

Answer: (a)   Percutaneous nephrolithotripsy (PCNL) can be effectively used to extract large stones in the pediatric population. Though renal parenchymal bleeding can occur, only the use of an access tract <22F is associated with a decreased risk of transfusion. Multiple access tracts may be necessary and have not been shown to increase the risk of transfusion.

Renal parenchymal imaging in children

27

Jason W Anast and Paul F Austin

(Based on chapter by J Michael Zerin)

1. Which of the following is the *least* sensitive test for diagnosing pyelonephritis?

   (a) DMSA
   (b) Ultrasound
   (c) Computerized tomography (CT)
   (d) Magnetic resonance imaging (MRI)

   Answer: (b) DMSA, CT, and MRI all have sensitivity >90% for diagnosing pyelonephritis. While renal ultrasound is often ordered in patients with suspected pyelonephritis, subtle changes in parenchymal echogenicity are often difficult to differentiate. Additionally, purulent urine can be difficult to differentiate sonographically from desquamated cellular material in a chronically obstructed, uninfected system.

2. Which of the following is *true* regarding renal vein thrombosis in children?

   (a) CT and MRI are useful imaging tests for diagnosing renal vein thrombosis
   (b) The classic presentation of renal vein thrombosis is gross hematuria, hypotension, and an enlarged, palpable kidney
   (c) Risk factors for renal vein thrombosis include prematurity, mother with diabetes, severe dehydration, sepsis, or coagulopathy
   (d) In the chronic phase of renal vein thrombosis, the kidney becomes enlarged on ultrasound with decreased echogenicity
   (e) In the acute phase of renal vein thrombosis, MAG3 renal scintography reveals a markedly enlarged kidney with increased uptake and no excretion

   Answer: (c) CT and MRI are rarely performed in children since renal vein thrombosis can usually be easily diagnosed with ultrasound or MAG3 renal scintigraphy. The classic presentation of renal vein thrombosis is gross hematuria, hypertension, and an enlarged, palpable kidney. In the acute phase, the kidney is enlarged, the parenchyma is diffusely echogenic on ultrasound, and MAG3 scintigraphy revealed reduced or absent uptake with no excretion of the tracer. In the chronic phase, renal function diminishes and the kidney becomes small and remains echogenic, and calcifications may appear within thrombosed intrarenal veins.

3. Which of the following is *not* true regarding imaging in Wilms' tumor?

   (a) The ultrasound appearance is usually a solid, hyperechoic renal mass
   (b) The CT appearance is usually a low attenuation before contrast and variable enhancement on postcontrast scans
   (c) Postnephrectomy surveillance is usually performed with ultrasound of the surgical bed and of the contralateral kidney

(d) CT and MRI generally provide the same information about tumor extent and are superior to ultrasound for tumor staging

(e) Ultrasound and MRI are generally more sensitive than CT at identifying renal vein and inferior vena cava (IVC) thrombus

Answer: (e) The ultrasound appearance of Wilms' tumor typically demonstrates a solid, hyperechoic renal mass, while CT imaging usually reveals a low-attenuation solid mass prior to contrast and variable enhancement postcontrast. MRI typically shows a low signal renal mass on T1-weighted sequences and a bright solid mass on T2 images. In general, CT and MRI provide more accurate tumor staging than ultrasound. CT and MRI are also more accurate than ultrasound for detecting renal vein and IVC tumor thrombus. Postnephrectomy, Doppler ultrasound is usually utilized for routine surveillance and can aid in identifying small masses.

4. Which of the following is *true* about imaging of malignant renal tumors in children?

(a) Malignant rhabdoid tumor is an aggressive, infiltrating renal tumor which can be detected with ultrasound, MRI, or CT, and usually arises in the parenchyma with invasion into the renal hilum

(b) Clear cell sarcoma is usually a solid, complex mass on ultrasound, CT, or MRI, with an appearance usually distinguishable from Wilms' tumor

(c) Renal medullary carcinoma is a very aggressive tumor, with minimal enhancement on CT or MRI

(d) The imaging characteristics of renal cell carcinoma in children are similar to those in adults, with the tumor appearing hyperechoic on ultrasound and hyperdense on CT

(e) In leukemia and lymphoma, renal involvement is usually unilateral, with tumors appearing as distinct masses on ultrasound

Answer: (d) Malignant rhabdoid tumor is an aggressive neoplasm which usually arises from the renal hilum and may extend into the parenchyma. Clear cell sarcoma is usually indistinguishable from Wilms' tumor on abdominal imaging. Renal medullary carcinoma is a very aggressive tumor, with heterogeneous enhancement on CT and MRI. The appearance of renal cell carcinoma in children is similar to that in adults, with the tumor appearing hyperechoic on ultrasound and hyperdense on CT. In leukemia and lymphoma, renal involvement is usually bilateral, with leukemic infiltrates presenting as diffuse renal enlargement with disruption of the normal corticomeduallary junction, and lymphocytic infiltrates presenting as nonspecific renal enlargement with diffuse increase in parenchymal echogenicity on ultrasound.

5. A 3-week-old boy is noted to have an enlarged right kidney with multiple cysts of varying sizes on abdominal ultrasound. A MAG3 renal scan reveals 3% function of the right kidney. What is the most likely diagnosis?

(a) Multicystic dysplastic kidney
(b) Autosomal recessive polycystic kidney disease
(c) Autosomal dominant polycystic kidney disease
(d) Multilocular cystic nephroma
(e) Juvenile nephronophthisis

Answer: (a) The description of a kidney with multiple cysts of varying sizes with minimal or no function is characteristic of multicystic dysplastic kidney. Autosomal recessive polycystic kidney disease presents as enlarged and echogenic kidneys. Autosomal dominant polycystic kidney disease usually demonstrates a functioning kidney with few small cysts early in life that enlarge throughout childhood and adulthood. Multilocular cystic nephroma is a benign condition that presents as a complex, multilocular mass within the kidney. Juvenile nephronophthisis is an autosomal recessive disorder characterized by kidneys with increased echogenicity, with microscopic medullary cysts that gradually develop into visible larger cysts.

Assessment of renal obstructive disorders: ultrasound, nuclear medicine, and magnetic resonance imaging

28

James Elmore and Andrew J Kirsch

1. A 3-year-old girl is found to have bilateral SFU (Society of Fetal Urology) grade 3 hydronephrosis during a work-up for a febrile urinary tract infection (UTI). A voiding cystourethrogram (VCUG) is performed and is negative. The best study to determine differential renal function, the degree of obstruction, and to assess for a crossing vessel is:

   (a) Renal ultrasound
   (b) Computerized tomography (CT) abdomen and pelvis with contrast
   (c) MAG3 renal scan
   (d) Gadolinium enhanced magnetic resonance imaging (MRI)

   Answer: (d) Rationale: Although all of these studies would provide important information in this case, none except for MRI provides differential function, assesses the degree of obstruction, and provides the anatomical detail needed to see a crossing vessel.

2. All of the following are reasons that ultrasonography is a useful screening tool for the evaluation of a child with a history of a febrile UTI *except*:

   (a) It provides functional information
   (b) There is no exposure to radiation
   (c) It is inexpensive
   (d) It is readily available

   Answer: (a) Rationale: Ultrasonography is a useful screening tool because it is inexpensive, readily available, and does not use radiation. Ultrasonography does not provide functional information.

3. The radiopharmaceutical that is 90% bound to plasma proteins and is principally cleared by tubular secretion is:

   (a) Tc-Mercaptoacetyltriglycine (MAG3)
   (b) Tc-Diethylenetriaminepentaacetic (DTPA)
   (c) Tc-Dimercaptosuccinic acid (DMSA)
   (d) Tc-Glycerinaldehydic acid (GAA)

   Answer: (a) Rationale: Tc-MAG3 is primarily bound to plasma proteins and is cleared by tubular secretion. Tc-DTPA is cleared by glomerular filtration. Tc-DMSA is unique in that it tightly binds the renal tubular cells and very little is excreted in the urine. These properties make each useful in different scenarios.

4. The renal handling of gadolinium-DTPA (Gd-DTPA) during MR urography is determined by the:

   (a) Gadolinium
   (b) DTPA

(c) The ratio of gadolinium to DTPA

(d) Creatinine clearance

Answer: (b) Rationale: DTPA is handled identically by the kidney whether it is attached to radionuclide or to a contrast agent.

5. A major disadvantage to performing MR urography in children is:

    (a) The use of ionizing radiation

    (b) Adverse biological long-term effects

    (c) Restricted use to normal renal function

    (d) The need for sedation or anesthesia

Answer: (d) Rationale: The major disadvantages of MR urography are the need for sedation in children younger than about 5 years of age and the cost.

6. A boy with a functionally solitary kidney is diagnosed with SFU grade 2–3 hydronephrosis. The main advantage of obtaining an MR urogram in comparison to more conventional imaging modalities (i.e. diuretic renography) is:

    (a) The low cost of the imaging study

    (b) Accurate functional data even in poorly functioning renal units

    (c) Gadolinium never causes allergic reactions

    (d) Acquisition of anatomic and functional data in a single study

Answer: (d) Rationale: MR urography offers both functional and anatomical information which equals or surpasses that obtained with any other imaging modality. Answer (b) is also true but not the principal advantage in this scenario.

7. A patient with myelodysplasia is referred for MR urography. The presence of potentially harmful ferromagnetic implants:

    (a) Will be evaluated by the radiologist

    (b) Can be neglected due to compensatory MR settings

    (c) Needs to be evaluated by the referring physician

    (d) New implants are all MR compatible

Answer: (c) Rationale: The physician ordering any radiographic study should be aware of potential contraindications. Metallic implants are a contraindication to MR urography and these patients should undergo alternative studies.

8. A patient with left flank pain is evaluated by Doppler ultrasonography. During the study a resistive index (RI) is calculated. Regarding the RI, urinary obstruction would be suggested by all of the following except:

    (a) An interrenal RI difference >0.10

    (b) An abnormal RI response to a diuretic challenge

    (c) An RI >0.7

    (d) A relatively high diastolic flow compared to systolic flow

Answer: (d) Rationale: A high RI index (>0.7) is suggestive of obstruction. Since the RI is based on the ratio of diastolic flow to systolic flow, increasing diastolic flow reduces the RI and is therefore not suggestive of obstruction.

Assessment of renal obstructive disorders: urodynamics of the upper tract

29

Thomas E Novak and Yegappan Lakshmanan

1. In the evaluation of hydronephrosis, upper tract infusion pressure/flow studies differ from nuclear renal scans and sonograms in their measurement of:

   (a) Outflow resistance
   (b) Renal blood flow
   (c) Glomerular filtration rate
   (d) Degree of dilation

   Answer: (a) In any biological fluid conduit system, the resistance of the conduit is directly proportional to pressure/flow. Both pressure and flow must be accounted for in the measurement of resistance. (Page 461)

2. Animal models and human studies suggest that undesirable physiologic renal changes begin to take place above what pelvic pressure?

   (a) $10\,cmH_2O$
   (b) $14\,cmH_2O$
   (c) $18\,cmH_2O$
   (d) $22\,cmH_2O$

   Answer: (b) Although the exact precise threshold pressure above which renal injury occurs is not known, studies in rats and pigs suggest that this number lies between 10 and $20\,cmH_2O$. In humans, the intrarenal arterial pressure rises acutely above renal pelvic pressures of $14\,cmH_2O$. Based on these observations, $14\,cmH_2O$ has been accepted as the upper threshold for normal renal pelvic pressure. (Page 463)

3. When using upper tract pressure/flow studies in children, consideration for which of the following parameters allows for a more meaningful interpretation:

   (a) Maximum physiologic urine output
   (b) Presence of microscopic hematuria
   (c) Calculation of renal blood flow
   (d) Detrusor leak point pressure

   Answer: (a) A limitation of the initial infusion pressure/flow study as described by Whitaker is that infusion rates did not account for the age and size of a child. One can estimate a patient's maximum physiologic urine output based on the 90th percentile glomerular filtration rate (GFR) for their body surface area (available in nomograms). The equation given on page 464 assumes that under nonpathologic conditions, maximum diuresis is 20% of the GFR. This calculation allows the urologist to individually tailor infusion rates based on the age and size of the child. (Page 463)

4. An 8-year-old girl has ongoing intermittent right-sided abdominal pain, nausea and emesis 1 year following pyeloplasty for uretero-pelvic junction obstruction (UPJO). A sonogram demonstrates residual hydronephrosis of the

right kidney with mild cortical thinning. The left kidney is normal. On diuretic renography, the right kidney clears after administration of furosemide at T1/2 = 18 min (indeterminate range). An infusion pressure flow study of the right kidney is performed. The maximum renal pelvic pressure following administration of furosemide is 10 cmH$_2$O. The next step is:

(a) Termination of study
(b) Drainage of the bladder
(c) Individualized infusion pressure-flow study
(d) Antegrade nephrostogram

Answer: (c) Infusion pressure/flow studies are useful in the evaluation of postsurgical upper tract dilation. Renal pelvic pressures >14 cmH$_2$O during the diuresis pressure-flow portion of the study are indicative of obstruction. In that event, an antegrade nephrostogram is performed and study is concluded. If the pressure does not exceed 14 cmH$_2$O during diuresis, an individualized infusion pressure-flow study should be performed. (Page 473)

5. The ureteral opening pressure is defined as:

(a) The difference calculated between the bladder pressure and renal pelvic pressure during maximum infusion
(b) The renal pelvic pressure at which contrast is first visualized in the ureter under fluoroscopy
(c) The renal pelvic pressure measured immediately after introduction of the transducer into the renal pelvis

(d) The renal pelvic pressure subtracted from the abdominal pressure

Answer: (b) Periodic fluoroscopic monitoring is an important part of infusion pressure-flow studies of the kidney. The presence of a ureteral opening pressure of >14 cmH$_2$O is strongly predictive of a positive individualized pressure-flow study. (Page 470)

6. Patients with a positive infusion pressure-flow study of the upper tract should:

(a) Have the ureter stented while under anesthesia
(b) Maintain the urethral catheter for 1 week prior to removal
(c) Undergo diuretic Doppler sonography with calculation of the resistive index
(d) Be placed on oral prophylactic antibiotics until definitive correction

Answer: (d) One of the disadvantages of infusion pressure-flow studies of the upper tract is that they are invasive. Infection is a possible complication and this can be especially troublesome in an obstructed kidney. Routine preprocedural urine culture and prophylactic antibiotics prior to introduction of the needle are recommended. Patients with a positive examination should remain on a prophylactic dose of oral antibiotics until definitive surgical correction. (Page 473)

Reference

1. Whitaker RH. Diagnosis of obstruction in dilated ureters. Ann R Coll Surg Engl 1973; 53: 153–66.

Ureteropelvic junction obstruction and multicystic dysplastic kidney: surgical management

30

Michael C Carr

1. In a 6-week-old infant who has <10% function to a kidney with a radiographically diagnosed ureteropelvic junction obstruction, appropriate options for their management would be all of the following except:

    (a) Temporary nephrostomy tube drainage
    (b) Placement of double stent for 4–6 weeks with repeat renal scan to assess for improved function
    (c) Dismembered pyeloplasty and double stent placement at time of surgery
    (d) Laparoscopic retroperitoneal dismembered pyeloplasty
    (e) Nephrectomy if cortical cysts are encountered at the time of exploration

    Answer: (d) Temporary drainage may differentiate those kidneys that have recoverable function from those that have irreversible injury or renal dysplasia and/or hypoplasia. Early surgery may allow for an easier repair than one in which a double J stent or a nephrostomy tube causes trauma to the renal pelvis. The presence of cortical cysts generally correlates with diffuse glomerulosclerosis. Laparoscopic surgery is a viable option but the technical nuances in a 6-week-old infant preclude its use.

2. A ureteropelvic junction obstruction in which there is a 4 cm narrowing of the proximal

ureter along with a very generous renal pelvis can be optimally managed with which repair:

    (a) Foley Y-V plasty
    (b) Davis intubated ureterotomy
    (c) Scardino-Prince vertical flap pyeloureteroplasty
    (d) Anderson-Hynes dismembered pyeloplasty
    (e) Retrograde endopyelotomy

    Answer: (c) The Scardino-Prince vertical flap can be fashioned to provide a long flap which can be fashioned even onto the posterior aspect of the renal pelvis. In doing so, even a ureteral narrowing of several centimeters can be overcome. A Foley Y-V plasty would work for only limited length; an intubated ureterotomy would be similar in use to an endopyelotomy and is generally not a good choice for longer narrowed ureters. A dismembered pyeloplasty may be limiting if the ureter and/or kidney cannot be mobilized to provide for a tension-free anastomosis.

3. Repairs of an infant's ureteropelvic junction obstruction should involve all of the following except:

    (a) Judicious handling of tissues and use of traction sutures
    (b) Either internal stenting with a double J stent or nephrostomy tube, or placement

of a Penrose drain without internal stenting

(c) Aggressive reduction of the renal pelvis prior to completing a dismembered pyeloplasty

(d) A running or interrupted closure with eversion of the mucosa to provide for a watertight anastomosis

Answer: (c) The technical aspects in performing an infant pyeloplasty amount to minimizing tissue trauma to decrease postoperative edema and potential devascularization. Aggressive reduction of the renal pelvis risks inadvertent infundibular injury. Creation of a funnel-shaped dependent tension-free anastomosis is the most important objective.

4. A multicystic kidney which fails to involute over a period of several years may warrant surgical removal due to the risk of malignancy or future hypertension, albeit very rare. Optimal surgical management in an 8-year-old child with a noninvoluting 7 cm multicystic dysplastic kidney would be:

(a) Anterior subcostal open nephrectomy
(b) Laparoscopic nephrectomy
(c) Flank incision and open nephrectomy
(d) Posterior lumbotomy and nephrectomy

Answer: (b) Surgical removal of a multicystic dysplastic kidney has been accomplished readily through any number of incisions.

The advent of laparoscopy with 5 mm instruments allows for easy, safe removal of a kidney with minimal morbidity giving the best cosmetic outcome and thus would be the favored approach.

5. In the case of a redo pyeloplasty in a 3-year-old child in which there was known to be urinary extravasation postoperatively along with aggressive tailoring of the renal pelvis, the preferred approach to the repair would be:

(a) A redo open dismembered pyeloplasty
(b) A laparoscopic dismembered pyeloplasty
(c) A retrograde endopyelotomy with laser
(d) A ureterocalicostomy with amputation of the lower pole parenchyma
(e) Antegrade Acucize endopyelotomy

Answer: (d) The anatomy of the persistent ureteropelvic junction obstruction will dictate the repair, but significant urinary extravasation and aggressive tailoring of the renal pelvis will make a dismembered pyeloplasty difficult, either open or laparoscopically. A ureterocalicostomy, in which there is already thinning of the lower pole parenchyma and a dilated calyx, should provide the most durable long-term outcome. A focal stenosis in which the anastomosis was in a dependent position may lend itself to an endopyelotomy, either antegrade or retrograde, depending on the patient's age.

Laparoscopic nephrectomy and pyeloplasty

31

CD Anthony Herndon
(Based on chapter by Alaa El-Ghoneimi)

1. For the laparoscopic lateral retroperitoneal approach for nephrectomy, which attachment should be taken down last:

   (a) Posterior
   (b) Inferior
   (c) Anterior
   (d) Superior
   (e) Lateral

   Answer: (c) With the retroperitoneal approach, the anterior surface of the kidney should be dissected last. It serves as an anchor to keep the kidney reflected anteriorly, and allows for easy identification of the hilar vessels and ureter posteriorly as they lie on the psoas muscle which is the posterior limit of dissection.

2. For the lateral retroperitoneal pyeloplasty, which is identified upon first entry into the retroperitoneum:

   (a) Aorta
   (b) Renal artery
   (c) Renal vein
   (d) Renal pelvis
   (e) Adrenal gland

   Answer: (b) The renal artery lies most posterior, during retroperitoneal access it should be visualized first. The renal vein is above this and the renal pelvis sits most anterior. If a renal artery is seen anterior to the ureter during this approach, then it represents a crossing vessel and the repair should be performed while reflecting this lower pole vessel posteriorly.

3. In which approach is it necessary to mobilize the colon prior to laparoscopic renal surgery?

   (a) Right lateral retroperitoneal
   (b) Left transperitoneal
   (c) Left lateral retroperitoneal
   (d) Right transperitoneal
   (e) Prone retroperitoneal

   Answer: (d) Mobilization of the colon is usually required for transperitoneal right renal surgery. The transmesenteric approach is not ideal and typically is impeded by the duodenum or vena cava. By mobilizing the colon, the Kocher maneuver can be avoided and excellent exposure for the renal hilum and renal pelvis can be achieved.

Wilms' tumor

32

Sarah Marietti and Fernando Ferrer

(Based on chapter by Michael Ritchey and Fernando Ferrer)

1. All of the following syndromes are associated with Wilms' tumors except:

   (a) Wilms', aniridia, genital anomaly, mental retardation (WAGR) syndrome
   (b) Denys-Drash syndrome
   (c) Coloboma of the eye, heart defects, atresia of the choanae, retardation of growth and/or development, genital and/or urinary abnormalities, and ear abnormalities and deafness (CHARGE) syndrome
   (d) Soto's syndrome
   (e) Beckwith-Wiedemann syndrome (BWS)

   Answer: (c) 1% of Wilms' tumor patients are afflicted with the WAGR syndrome. Denys-Drash syndrome consists of mesangial sclerosis, pseudohermaphroditism and Wilms's tumors. There have been reports of Wilms' tumors associated with Soto's syndrome. The syndrome consists of excessive growth in the first 2 years of life, mental retardation, hypotonia and speech impairment. Patients with BWS have an incidence of Wilms' tumor of 10–20%. CHARGE syndrome consists of failure of ability to close the eye, heart defects, blocked nasal passages, mental retardation, underdeveloped sexual organs and ear abnormalities. This syndrome is not associated with Wilms' tumors.

2. Which of the following is true regarding the WT1 gene?

   (a) Is necessary for normal genitourinary development
   (b) Mutations are associated with Wilms' tumor 90% of the time
   (c) Is located on chromosome 11p13
   (d) Mutations are associated with blastemal pathology

   Answer: (c) The WT1 gene is located on 11p13 of chromosome 11 and is responsible for normal genitourinary development. Mutations have been attributed to extensive genitourinary defects including pseudohermaphroditism. Wilms' tumors are associated with mutations of the WT1 gene <10% of the time. Germline mutations have been found in familial Wilms' tumors, and when present are associated with a predominant stromal pathology. A WT1 mutation is rarely found in the Wilms' tumor patient without a specific syndrome or genitourinary anomaly.

3. Unfavorable histology:

   (a) Is present in 50% of Wilms' tumors
   (b) Is defined by large polyploid nuclei
   (c) Is most commonly present in the first 2 years of life
   (d) Is associated with resistance to chemotherapy

   Answer: (d) Unfavorable histology is associated with increased rates of relapse and death. This histology is present in approximately 10% of Wilms' tumors, but responsible for over 50% of deaths from Wilms' tumors. It is defined by large polyploid nuclei and is rare in the first 2 years of life, however, in children over 5 years of age the incidence increases to 13%. It is associated with resistance to chemotherapy and can be divided into focal or diffuse patterns. When all anaplastic components are removed outcomes are still very good. Thus, unfavorable histology is not a marker for aggressiveness of the tumor, but predominantly a marker for chemoresistance.

4. According to data obtained from National Wilms' Tumor (NWTS) and Children's Oncology Group (COG) renal tumor studies, which statement is true?

    (a) Stage I and II favorable histology tumors should be treated with radiation
    (b) Stage IV favorable histology disease treated with vincristine, dactinomycin, doxorubicin and cyclophosphamide have significant improvement in survival
    (c) Risk of death for stage III and IV favorable histology increased with loss of heterozygosity for chromosome 16q and 1p
    (d) The presence of lymph node metastasis does not negatively affect prognosis

Answer: (c) The NWTS-3 demonstrated that children with favorable histology stage I and II tumors treated with vincristine, dactinomycin and radiation did no better than those whose radiation was omitted with overall survival rates reaching 91%. They also demonstrated that patients with stage IV favorable histology treated with dactinomycin, vincristine, doxorubicin and cyclophosphamide did no better than those treated with only the three drugs dactinomycin, vincristine and doxorubicin. Thus, the use of cyclophosphamide was omitted for this group. NWTS-5 was a single-arm therapeutic trial designed to collect information about the biologic features of the tumors. They found that loss of heterozygosity for both 16q and 1p increased the risk of relapse and death

for patients with stage III and IV favorable histology. These markers can be used as independent prognostic factors.

5. Complications of chemotherapy include all of the following except:

    (a) Doxorubicin use increases the chance of developing secondary malignancy
    (b) Alkylating agents can chronically damage germ cell production in both the pre- and postpubertal testis
    (c) Congestive heart failure is a known complication of vincristine treatment
    (d) Growth disturbance is a direct effect of spinal irradiation and chemotherapeutic effects on chondrocytes

Answer: (c) Children treated with Wilms' tumors are at increased risk for developing second malignant neoplasms. The risk of leukemia or lymphoma is greatest in the 8 years following treatment, but the risk of solid tumors continues to rise as the child gets older. The use of doxorubicin has been associated with increased risk of second malignancy. Doxorubicin is also cardiotoxic and is associated with increased risk of congestive heart failure, the risk is proportional to the dose of doxorubicin received. Alkylating agents have been found to damage germ cells at all ages, although prior reports believed that the prepubertal testis was resistant to chronic toxicity. Growth disturbances occur as a direct result of chondrocyte damage. The reduction in height is a direct result of amount of radiation, however, with the current radiation doses given, the effect should not be clinically apparent.

6. The best test to detect inferior vena cava thrombosis and extent is:

    (a) Computerized tomography (CT) scan with contrast

(b) Ultrasound
(c) Magnetic resonance imaging (MRI)
(d) CT scan without contrast

Answer: (c) Caval thrombus may be visible on CT scan with intravenous contrast; however, the determination of extent of thrombus is best visualized with MRI. Ultrasound may also be used to evaluate for presence or absence of thrombus, but precision is limited in demonstrating exact anatomical location and extent.

Surgical approaches for renal tumors 33

João L Pippi Salle, Armando J Lorenzo, and
Elizabeth R Williams

(Based on original chapter by JL Pippi Salle and Roman Jednak)

1. Which one of the following is not a beneficial effect of a mannitol when used in the surgical management of renal tumors?

   (a) Increases renal plasma flow
   (b) Minimizes cellular edema
   (c) Increases intravascular resistance
   (d) Promotes osmotic diuresis
   (e) None of the above

   Answer: (c) Mannitol is a drug commonly used in the management of renal tumors, particularly in partial nephrectomies. There are several potential benefits from using it, including stimulation of diuresis, decrease in cellular edema, and increase in renal plasma flow. Experimental evidence indicates that mannitol induces a decrease in renal intravascular resistance.

2. For renal tumors in which thrombus invasion involves the inferior vena cava, which of the following statements best reflects good surgical management?

   (a) Resection of the involved segment of the vena cava should be avoided at all cost, even if it includes leaving small amounts of residual tissue in the vessel wall
   (b) Right-sided renal tumors with involvement of vena cava cannot undergo supra renal resection of the inferior vena cava due to the risk of venous congestion of the left kidney
   (c) Computerized tomography (CT) scan of the abdomen and pelvis as an imaging study is enough in order to fully evaluate the presence and extension of an inferior vena cava tumor thrombus
   (d) Left-sided renal tumors pose a difficult challenge when associated with an inferior vena cava thrombus as supra renal resection of the inferior renal cava without reestablishment of caval venous flow may result in overwhelming venous congestion of residual right kidney
   (e) All of the above are important surgical issues to consider in this step of management of tumors

   Answer: (d) Involvement of the inferior vena cava poses a difficult challenge. In patients with suprahepatic extension preoperative chemotherapy is advised. In order to define the level of thrombus involvement preoperatively, Doppler ultrasound (including transesophageal echo) and/or magnetic resonance imaging (MRI) are obtained in those patients in whom there is clinical or radiological suspicion of involvement. A CT scan is somewhat limited in the evaluation of this problem. In patients who undergo surgical exploration, evidence of involvement of the vena caval wall indicates surgical resection whenever possible. If a large segment of vena cava is resected, the blood supply to the contralateral kidney may be compromised. Due to the large network of collaterals which the left kidney commonly has (i.e. gonadal, adrenal and lumbar veins as tributaries to the renal vein), obstruction of caval blood flow after resection of a right renal tumor is tolerated. On the contrary, the right kidney has poor collateral venous drainage, and may not fare well after resection of a left-sided renal mass with caval thrombus. Thus, in such cases, reconstruction of the vena cava to avoid overwhelming venous congestion of the right kidney is paramount.

3. In the management of renal masses in children, which of the following statements regarding partial nephrectomy is true?

   (a) Partial nephrectomy is the surgical approach of choice for all unilateral renal masses in children, as the goal is to preserve renal mass even if the risk of local recurrence is slightly higher
   (b) Patients with a bilateral Wilms' tumor benefit from partial nephrectomy prior to chemotherapy
   (c) Partial nephrectomy plays a role in the management of a patient with Wilms' tumor associated with Beckwith-Wiedemann syndrome or Wilms', aniridia, genital anomaly, mental retardation (WAGR) syndrome
   (d) Patients with biopsy-proven renal cell carcinoma should undergo immunotherapy or chemotherapy protocols prior to attempting partial nephrectomy
   (e) The prognosis of renal cell carcinoma after partial nephrectomy in children is equal to that of adults with similar stage of disease

Answer: (c) Partial nephrectomy is offered in selected cases in children with Wilms' tumors. Currently, protocols support its use in children with bilateral tumors or tumors involving a solitary kidney after chemotherapy. Also, it is advocated for children with syndromes that put them at high risk for metachronous ipsilateral and contralateral disease. Renal cell carcinoma is rare in children and appears to have a more favorable course than in adults. The data for partial nephrectomy in pediatric renal cell carcinoma are limited. There is no evidence that preoperative immunotherapy improves survival or facilitates surgical resection. Furthermore, experience in adult patients would suggest that cytoreductive surgery (i.e. tumor removal prior to systemic therapy) may be of benefit in some patients.

4. Regarding the management of congenital mesoblastic nephroma, which of the following statement(s) is/are false?

   (a) Congenital mesoblastic nephroma is one of the most common solid renal tumors in infancy
   (b) Partial nephrectomy is the treatment of choice for congenital mesoblastic nephroma
   (c) There is a small but real risk of local reoccurrence in patients with a cellular variant of congenital mesoblastic nephroma
   (d) Dissection of the renal hilum is particularly important as this site is the most common location for invasion and local reoccurrence
   (e) All of the above statements are true

Answer: (b) Congenital mesoblastic nephroma represents the most common solid renal mass in infants, particularly in the first 6 months of life. The treatment of choice is nephrectomy as the risk of residual disease is an important problem, particularly in those patients with the cellular variant of the tumor. The renal hilum dissection is also of crucial importance, where attention must be paid to complete removal of the tumor.

5. Which of the following are true danger points to be particularly considered in the resection of large renal masses in children?

   (a) A transmesenteric approach is preferred as it provides better exposure of the renal vessels as they enter the aorta and the vena cava
   (b) Great care should be paid to identify and avoid ligation of the superior mesenteric artery when exposure of left renal masses is attempted
   (c) Dissection of the renal hilum should be performed after complete mobilization of the kidney in order to allow proper exposure of the vessels in most cases
   (d) The renal vein is longer on the right side, therefore more easily controlled
   (e) Early ligation of the ureter is recommended in order to allow exposure and mobilization along the medial aspect of the kidney towards the renal hilum

Answer: (b)   Although an uncommon occurrence, dissection of the superior mesenteric artery can be carried out by mistakenly identifying it as the left renal artery. This can be seen in cases with large masses and displacement of the aorta. Keeping this danger point in mind is of crucial importance, as ligation of the superior mesenteric artery can lead to fatal complications (mesenteric ischemia). The approach to most renal masses is not transmesenteric; the colon should be reflected medially after incision of the Line of Toldt. It is advocated that the renal hilum should be controlled prior to complete mobilization in order to decrease the chance of tumor cells accessing the vascular system during aggressive manipulation. Furthermore, by securing the renal artery early, the tumor may be easier to dissect out and remove. Admittedly, this can not be done in all cases and some tumors need to by completely dissected in order to gain access to the renal artery from a posterior approach. The ureter should not be ligated and transected until the tumor is considered resectable. If early transection of the ureter is carried out and the tumor cannot be removed, the risk of postoperative obstruction or urine leak is increased.

6. Regarding tumor rupture and/or spillage, which of the following statements is false?

   (a) Preoperative chemotherapy increases the risk of tumor rupture with manipulation
   (b) Rupture of the renal capsule or presence of tumor spillage will upgrade the tumor stage of the kidney
   (c) Gerota's fascia should be removed with the kidney in order to try to minimize the chances of leaving residual microscopic disease behind, and decrease the chances of rupture
   (d) Peritoneal soiling is currently considered a stage 3, which adds radiation and chemotherapy to the management of these children
   (e) Bloody peritoneal fluid is a sign of major spillage

Answer: (a)   Tumor rupture or spillage is of great concern. Due to the increased risk of local recurrence, it calls for more aggressive management including radiation. Consequently, it increases the stage. Evidence of peritoneal soiling – either by detection of peritoneal implants or the presence of bloody peritoneal fluid – is considered diffuse soiling (not limited to the retroperitoneum). Preoperative chemotherapy in general makes the tumors less friable and potentially decreases the chances of tumor rupture.

7. Regarding the arterial vascularization of the kidney, which of the following statements is true?

   (a) There are no defined vascularized segments and the vascular supply is extremely variable between patients

(b) Multiple renal arteries occur in up to 23% of patients

(c) Ligation of a branch of the renal arteries is of no consequence due to the rich collateral blood supply of the kidney

(d) Warm ischemia by temporary occlusion of the renal artery can be safely tolerated for >1 h without any important consequences for renal function

(e) All of the above statements are true

Answer: (b)   Multiple renal arteries are not uncommonly seen. Up to 23% of patients have multiple arteries in one kidney. The arterial blood supply to the kidney has well-defined segments and is devoid of collaterals. Therefore, ligation of a branch leads to ischemia of the segment it supplies. Warm ischemia is not well tolerated. After 30 min of warm vascular occlusion the progression of ischemic cellular damage increases. Therefore, cooling the kidney is an important maneuver to exercise in prolonged partial resections.

8. In regards to the surgical management of Wilms' tumors, the decision to call the tumor inoperable _____:

(a) Should be reached prior to surgery without exploration

(b) Intra-operative biopsy should be avoided at all costs in patients who are deemed inoperable and those children should undergo chemotherapy based on clinical characteristics

(c) A full lymph node dissection is required in patients that undergo a radical nephrectomy for Wilms' tumor

(d) A pathology specimen should be sent in formalin

(e) Surgical exploration is avoided for patients who have preoperative imaging consistent with bilateral disease and/or suprahepatic extension of tumor thrombus

Answer: (e)   Aside from children with bilateral tumors, tumors in a solitary kidney and

extensive tumor thrombus (i.e. above the hepatic veins), the decision to call a tumor inoperable should be finalized in the operating room (after exploration). In cases where the involvement of surrounding structures precludes safe resection, the tumor should be biopsied in order to have histological information prior to chemotherapy (following the Children's Oncology Group protocols). Lymph node sampling is wise to perform but a full lymph node dissection is not required. In general, pathology specimens should be sent fresh and not in formalin.

9. Which one of the following is the best surgical approach for a unilateral renal mass in a child who has not received previous chemotherapy?

(a) Retroperitoneal through a flank incision

(b) Retroperitoneal through a dorsal lumbotomy incision

(c) Transperitoneal through a subcostal or transverse abdominal incision

(d) Transperitoneal using a laparoscopic approach

(e) All of the above are acceptable options

Answer: (c)   The surgical approach of choice in children with possible Wilms' tumor is trasperitoneal, usually through a subcostal or transverse abdominal incision. The laparoscopic approach has been used in a few institutions after administration of chemotherapy (following the Society of Pediatric Oncology (SIPO) protocols favored in Europe and parts of South America). The retroperitoneal approach through a flank or dorsal lumbotomy incision leads to limited exposure in children and is generally avoided.

10. After hilar dissection during a partial nephrectomy, you are about to clamp the renal artery. Preparation to minimize the effects of ischemia includes all of the following except:

(a) Cooling the kidney with ice

(b) Generous hydration prior to clamping

(c) Simultaneously clamping both the artery and vein

(d) Administering mannitol prior to clamping

(e) Minimizing traction on the kidney during resection

Answer: (c)   Simultaneous occlusion of both vessels produces additional venous congestion and renal damage. All of the other maneuvers described above help to minimize the effects of ischemia on the kidney and are considered routine during nephron-sparing surgery.

11. While examining a patient with a known renal mass, which of the following findings is not consistent with intravascular tumor extension?

(a) Bilateral lower extremity edema

(b) Varicocele

(c) Dilated superficial abdominal veins

(d) Proteinuria

(e) Peripheral neuropathy

Answer: (e) Venous congestion due to tumor infiltration of the vascular system can manifest in a variety of ways. All of the choices above result from inferior vena cava (IVC) extension of tumor thrombus except for peripheral neuropathy. If any of these findings is discovered on exam, MRI or color Doppler ultrasonography is used to confirm the presence of intravascular extension.

12. A 13-month-old male undergoes a left nephrectomy and the pathology reveals rhabdoid tumor of the kidney. In addition to a hematology-oncology referral, which of the following should be ordered?

(a) Bone scan

(b) MRI of the head

(c) Duplex ultrasound of the lower extremities

(d) Transthoracic echocardiogram

Answer: (b)   The most common metastatic site for rhabdoid tumor of the kidney is the

brain. All patients with this diagnosis should undergo either a CT or MRI of the brain. Additional testing may be necessary, but none of the other tests listed are indicated in the absence of associated symptoms.

13. A 4-year-old girl presents with a right renal mass with no evidence of extension beyond the right kidney on preoperative imaging. During dissection of the mass off the adrenal, a 0.5 cm incidental incision is made into the renal capsule without evidence of gross tumor spillage and with careful avoidance of peritoneal contamination. On final pathology, the tumor is identified as a Wilms' tumor. The left kidney is uninvolved with tumor on inspection and there is no evidence of spread beyond the kidney. What is the final staging?

(a) Stage I

(b) Stage II

(c) Stage III

(d) Stage IV

(e) Stage V

Answer: (b)   The tumor is completely excised except for local tumor spillage into the flank when the capsule was violated. Tumor spillage into the peritoneum would have upgraded the case to a stage III.

14. Which of the following would not be an indication for partial nephrectomy for a Wilms' tumor?

(a) Solitary kidney

(b) Bilateral tumors

(c) Renal failure

(d) Beckwith-Wiedemann syndrome

(e) 2 cm tumor based on CT findings

Answer: (e)   Partial nephrectomy is not the standard of care for management of Wilms' tumors. However, there are situations in which partial nephrectomy is indicated. Partial nephrectomy is utilized in cases mandating nephron-sparing surgery (solitary kidney, bilateral masses, renal insufficiency) in order to minimize the risk of subsequent dialysis. Additionally, certain syndromes such as Beckwith-Wiedemann and WAGR predispose patients to developing Wilms' tumors. Partial nephrectomy is indicated since these patients have an increased likelihood of recurrent disease. Tumor size is not a criterion used during evaluation for partial nephrectomy.

15. After making a subcostal incision in a 6-year-old girl with a right renal mass suspicious for renal cell carcinoma, you note peritoneal metastases. Frozen section of one of these metastases reveals Wilms' tumor. Which of the following is not appropriate surgical technique?

    (a) Extend the surgical excision across the midline

    (b) Open Gerota's fascia and examine the contralateral kidney
    (c) Perform a lymph node sampling
    (d) Perform a partial nephrectomy
    (e) Perform a right radical nephrectomy with careful avoidance of tumor spillage

Answer: (d) When a Wilms' tumor is encountered intraoperatively, certain surgical modifications need to be implemented. The incision often needs to be extended in order to adequately assess for tumor in the contralateral kidney. A focused lymph node sampling should be performed, including any suspicious lymph nodes and nodes along the iliac, para-aortic, and celiac regions. A partial nephrectomy is not appropriate in the setting of normal renal function and no risk factors for recurrent Wilms' tumor.

Pediatric upper tract trauma

34

Douglas A Husmann

1. A patient that has gross hematuria disproportionate to the degree of trauma sustained suggests the finding of a:

   (a) Uretero-pelvic junction (UPJ) disruption
   (b) Intraperitoneal bladder rupture
   (c) Traumatic arterial-venous (AV) fistula formation
   (d) Thoracic or lumbar spinal fracture
   (e) Preexisting congenital renal anomaly

   Answer: (e)   The presence of gross hematuria disproportionate to the severity of the history of the traumatic injury classically suggests that a preexisting renal anomaly is present. Specifically, genitourinary (GU) anomalies found with this history in order of decreasing frequency are UPJ obstruction, hydrouretero-nephrosis (refluxing, obstructive or nonob-structive–nonrefluxing variants), and renal fusion anomalies (horseshoe kidneys). Approximately 30% of patients with UPJ disruption will have no degree of hematuria, with the vast majority of patients with a UPJ disruption having severe life-threatening associated injuries which resulted in inadequate radiographic staging studies being performed. The presence of multiple life-threatening injuries and the need for emergent life-saving surgery results in inadequate radiographic staging, leading to a missed or delayed diagnosis of the UPJ disruption in >50% of patients.

2. A single-phase computerized tomography (CT) scan obtained in the assessment of GU trauma is most likely to miss the majority of what type of injuries:

   (a) UPJ disruption
   (b) Grade 2 renal injury
   (c) Traumatic intimal renal artery disruption
   (d) Perinephric urinoma developing from a major renal laceration
   (e) Subcapsular hematomas which will cause a Page kidney affect (posttraumatic hypertension)

   Answer: (a)   A single-phase CT study is beneficial in determining renal perfusion, and will accurately diagnose renal artery intimal tears, grade 2 renal injuries and the presence of subcapsular hematomas. It may on occasion miss the presence of urinary extravasation developing as a consequence of a major renal laceration, it is however notoriously famous for missing the vast majority of isolated ureteral injuries and UPJ disruptions. A triphasic CT study (precontrast study, followed by a study immediately following injection and then a 15–20 min delayed study) is the most sensitive method for diagnosis and classification of renal trauma, and is highly accurate in diagnosing isolated ureteral injuries.

3. Following a traumatic injury a CT of the abdomen reveals a renal laceration that extends into 2 cm past the renal cortex, no urinary extravasation is seen. The injury is associated

with a devitalized renal fragment, the grade of renal injury is:

(a) 1
(b) 2
(c) 3
(d) 4
(e) 5

Answer: (c)

Grading of renal injuries

Grade of Renal Injury	Description
1	Renal contusion or subcapsular hematoma
2	Nonexpanding perirenal hematoma, <1 cm parenchymal laceration, no urinary extravasation, all renal fragments viable
3	Nonexpanding perirenal hematoma, >1 cm parenchymal laceration, no urinary extravasation, renal fragments may be viable or devitalized
4	Laceration extending into the collecting system with urinary extravasation, renal fragments may be viable or devitalized *or* Injury to the main renal vasculature with contained hemorrhage
5	Completely shattered kidney, by definition multiple major lacerations of >1 cm associated with multiple devitalized fragments *or* Injury to the main renal vasculature with uncontrolled hemorrhage, renal hilar avulsion

4. A 13-year-old boy sustained a grade 4 renal injury, secondary to a skiing accident 1 week ago. He has been managed nonoperatively. His urine has been grossly clear for the past 24 h and he is allowed to ambulate. You are contacted by the junior urology resident on the service that shortly after ambulation the urinary drainage bag filled with grossly bloody urine associated with clots. The patient's vital signs are stable, no orthostatic blood pressure (BP) changes are noted, and a stat hematocrit (Hct) reveals a 2 point decrease from prior values. Your next step is:

(a) Reassurance, continue activity and force fluids
(b) Recommend bed rest, increase intravenous (IV) fluids and serial Hct assessment
(c) Recommend bed rest, increase IV fluids and stat CT scan
(d) Recommend bed rest, increase IV fluids, emergent angiography
(e) Emergent surgical exploration

Answer: (d)   Approximately 25% of patients with a grade 3–4 renal trauma, managed in a nonoperative fashion, will have persistent or delayed hemorrhage. Classically, delayed hemorrhage will present 10–14 days postinjury but may occur up to 1 month after the insult. Delayed hemorrhage usually arises from the development of bleeding arteriovenous fistulas or ruptures of traumatic-induced pseudoaneurysms. The traumatic induced arterial-venous malformations (AVMs) will not spontaneously resolve and may be associated with life-threatening hemorrhage. Management should be by restriction of activity, increase IV fluids, and angiographic embolization of the bleeding site. Remember, in a child, shock and orthostatic BP changes may be one of the latter signs of severe bleeding. Delay in management of this serious complication places the child's life in jeopardy. Recurrence of gross hematuria with clots after their urine has grossly cleared is one of the key findings suggestive for the development of bleeding from an AV malformation or rupture of a vascular pseudoaneurysm. Patients with a history of recurrent gross hematuria with clots after their urine has grossly cleared should undergo urgent/emergent angiographic evaluation and embolization of the bleeding site.

5. A 9-year-old boy sustained a left major renal laceration associated with a perinephric urinoma. Three days postinjury a repeat CT scan confirms a major renal laceration with perinephric urinoma of approximately 5–6 cm in diameter, the left distal ureter is visualized, and the right kidney is normal. Your next step is:

(a) Continued observation
(b) Cystoscopy and left ureteral stent placement
(c) Left percutaneous nephrostomy tube placement
(d) Percutaneous drainage of left perinephric urinoma
(e) Cystoscopy, left ureteral stent placement, and percutaneous drainage of perinephric urinoma

Answer: (a) Approximately 75% of traumatic-induced urinomas will spontaneously resolve. Intervention should be considered only if there is persistent flank pain, adynamic ileus, and/or recurrent fevers suggestive of infection. In these patients endoscopic intervention with cystoscopy, retrograde pyelography, and ureteral stent placement is the preferred treatment. Although percutaneous nephrostomy tube placement and ureteral stent placement are equally efficacious, the major advantage of stent placement is quality of life during convalescence. A disadvantage of a ureteral stent is that both stent placement and removal require anesthesia in a small child. In addition, the small ureteral stent 4–5F used in small children may be obstructed by blood clots and fail to adequately drain the kidney, resulting in persistent urinoma. Percutaneous nephrostomy tube placement is preferred in a patient failing endoscopic management. In a patient whose medical condition precludes the use of general anesthesia, or in patients where a fair amount of blood clots exist in the renal pelvis, occlusion of the small ureteral stent is likely to occur.

6. A 6-year-old boy on IV prophylaxis with cephazolin undergoes angiographic embolization of a traumatic AV fistula associated with a grade 4 left traumatic renal injury. On the night of the embolization he spikes a temperature to 40°C. BP is stable. Physical examination reveals a tender left flank and the absence of bowel sounds, no rebound or indirect tenderness is found. His urine is grossly clear. You recommend acetaminophen, blood and urine cultures, and:

(a) Continued observation
(b) Change in antibiotic coverage to piperacillin and metronidazole
(c) Retroperitoneal/renal ultrasound
(d) CT of abdomen and aspiration of perinephric hematoma/urinoma
(e) Emergent surgical exploration and removal of necrotic tissue

Answer: (a) Postembolization syndrome is manifested by pyrexia up to 40°C, flank pain, and adynamic ileus. Symptoms should resolve within 4 days after the embolization. When pyrexia develops, blood and urine cultures to rule out bacterial seeding of the necrotic tissue are necessary. Consideration for a repeat CT scan with possible aspiration, culture, and drainage of a perinephric hematoma/urinoma should be given if febrile response persists for >96 h or if the patient's clinical course should rapidly worsen. No indications for altering antibiotics, the performance of a renal ultrasound or emergent surgical exploration are present in this patient.

7. A 2-year-old boy is a victim of child abuse, he was thrown across the room striking his left flank on the arm of a chair. A single-phase CT scan reveals a massive spleenic rupture, coexisting with a large liver laceration and hemoperitoneum, both kidneys are visualized. His vital signs are rapidly deteriorating and the child undergoes an emergent partial

heptectomy and spleenectomy. Perihepatic drains are noted to have >250 ml output per shift beginning the first postoperative day. Drain creatinine of 15 mg/dl is noted. CT scan reveals good bilateral renal perfusion, large left perinephric urinoma, no distal left ureter is seen. Contrast is seen in the right distal ureter. Vital signs and hematocrit are normal and stable. Your next step is:

(a) Continued observation
(b) Left percutaneous nephrostomy tube
(c) Cystoscopy, retrograde pyelogram, and stent placement
(d) Cystoscopy, retrograde pyelogram, and surgical exploration with primary ureteral repair
(e) Surgical exploration with primary repair

Answer: (d) The majority of patients sustaining a traumatic UPJ disruption will present with vascular instability resulting in minimal to no emergent preoperative imaging. This results in the average time from injury to diagnosis of a UPJ disruption of 36 h. Patients with this injury usually present with increased drainage from intraoperative drains, postoperative fever, ileus or flank pain. Classic findings on cystogram are a perinephric urinoma, the absence of renal parenchymal injuries, and nonvisualization of the ipsilateral ureter. A retrograde pyelogram is extremely helpful in delineating the injury. If the diagnosis is made within 5 days of the injury, and the patient is clinically stable, open surgical repair is preferred. If a delay in diagnosis of ≥6 days occurs, or if the patient is clinically unstable, a percutaneous nephrostomy tube may be placed with plans for delayed repair at 6–8 weeks postinjury. Predelayed repair, assessment of ipsilateral renal function, and antegrade and retrograde pyelograms can be performed to delineate the extent of the injury. Surgical alternatives for repair would be primary uretero-ureterostomy, ileal ureter, autotransplanatation or primary nephrectomy.

8. Recommendations for radiologic follow-up of a grade 2 renal injury are repeat CT scan:

(a) Only if a patient develops systemic or localized signs or symptoms
(b) At 2–3 days posttraumatic injury
(c) At 3–4 weeks posttraumatic injury
(d) At 3 months posttraumatic injury
(e) At 2–3 days postinjury and again at 3 months posttraumatic injury

Answer: (a) Follow-up renal imaging is not recommended for grade 1–2 renal injuries and for grade 3 lacerations where all fragments are viable. In patients with grade 3 renal lacerations associated with devitalized fragments, grade 4 and salvaged grade 5 renal injuries, a repeat CT scan with delayed images should be obtained 2–3 days following the traumatic insult. This study serves the purpose of assessing the extent of the hematoma/urinoma and will serve as a baseline evaluation in case secondary hemorrhage or infection should occur. An additional 3-month follow-up triphasic CT scan is obtained to verify resolution of any perinephric urinoma and to define the anatomic configuration of the residual functioning renal parenchyma. Irrespective of the grade of the injury, repeat imaging with a triphasic CT scan is recommended for patients with a history of renal trauma that have a persistent and/or increased fever, worsening flank pain, or persistent gross hematuria >72 h following the traumatic insult.

9. Retroperitoneal (renal) exploration is recommended when:

(a) A stab wound to the flank associated with a grade 2 renal injury
(b) A 22 caliber gunshot wound (GSW) resulting in a grade 2 renal injury
(c) A motor-vehicle accident (MVA) results in an isolated grade 3 renal injury with devitalized renal fragments
(d) A nonhemorrhagic, nonexpanding retroperitoneal mass found on surgical exploration following a GSW

(e) An MVA resulting in the need for emergent laparotomy due to vascular instability, retroperitoneal hemorrhage found on exploration

Answer: (e)

Consensus Recommendations for Management of Renal Trauma

Clinical findings and/or grade of renal injury	Recommended treatment
Grade 1 or 2 renal injury irrespective of traumatic etiology	Nonoperative
Isolated grade 3, 4, and hemodynamically stable grade 5 renal injuries	Nonoperative
Uncontrollable renal hemorrhage/vascular instability (usually grade 4 vascular or grade 5 injuries)	Absolute requirement for surgical intervention
Persistent or delayed hemorrhage not responding to angiographic embolization	Absolute requirement for surgical intervention
Expanding pulsatile retroperitoneal mass found on surgical exploration for coexisting intraabdominal injuries	Absolute requirement for surgical intervention (verify contralateral renal function prior to exploration)
Penetrating trauma, inadequate preoperative radiographic staging due to vascular instability of patient, retroperitoneal hemorrhage found on exploration	Retroperitoneal (renal) exploration recommended (verify contralateral renal function)
Blunt trauma, inadequate preoperative radiographic staging due to vascular instability of patient, retroperitoneal hemorrhage found on exploration	Retroperitoneal (renal) exploration recommended (verify contralateral renal function)
Blunt/penetrating trauma, radiographic screening studies reveal grade 3 with devitalized renal fragments, grade 4 or 5 renal injury, coexisting intraabdominal injuries, especially, duodenum, pancreas and colon	Retroperitoneal (renal) exploration with renorrhaphy and repair recommended

10. A 7-year-old boy is involved in a pedestrian MVA. A CT scan taken 1 h following trauma reveals no perfusion, and subsequently no function, of the left kidney; the right kidney is within normal limits. No associated intraabdominal injuries are noted. Vital signs are stable and hemoglobin is normal. Your next step is:

(a) Observation
(b) Angiography with stenting of left renal artery
(c) Angiographic infusion of streptokinase into left renal artery
(d) Systemic heparinization
(e) Surgical exploration

Answer: (a) In a patient sustaining renal arterial trauma, the clinical triad of hemodynamic instability, inadequate collateral blood flow, and warm ischemic time almost invariably results in the inability to salvage renal function. Due to this finding, no attempt to repair injuries to segmental renal vessels should be considered, and repair of the traumatically injured main renal artery is seldom if ever indicated if a normal contralateral kidney is present.

Reconstruction of the main renal artery following trauma is only a consideration in patients that are hemodynamically stable with an injury to a solitary kidney or in patients where bilateral renal arterial injuries are found. The infrequent exception to this rule is the presence of an incomplete arterial injury where perfusion to the kidney has been maintained by flow of blood through either the partially occluded main renal artery or via collateral vessels.

The ureter

35

Martin Kaefer

(Based on chapter by Cem Akbal and Martin Kaefer)

1. All of the following statements regarding ureteral embryology are true except:

   (a) The development of the ureter begins as an out pouching of the mesonephric duct termed the ureteric bud during the fourth week of gestation
   (b) Transient luminal obstruction of the ureter occurs with subsequent recanalization during the 7th week of gestation
   (c) As the ureter enters into the bladder its sole contribution to trigonal formation is at the level of the superficial trigone
   (d) The renin-angiotensin system appears to play a major role in ureteral development

   Answer: (c) As the ureter penetrates the bladder, its muscular layers disperse and contribute to formation of both the deep and superficial trigone. The outer layer melds into the detrusor in the upper part of the hiatus to form Waldeyer's sheath, which attaches the ureter to the bladder and is in continuity with the deep trigone. As the ureter makes its transition to an intramural location the muscle fibers take on a primarily longitudinal orientation and these fibers spread out to form the borders of the superficial trigone.

2. Which appears to play the most important role in ureteral peristalsis?

   (a) The parasympathetic nervous system
   (b) The sympathetic nervous system
   (c) Spontaneous electrical activity initiated by pacemaker cells in the renal pelvis and upper ureter
   (d) Innervation provided by peptidergic nerves (e.g. tachykinins, substance P)
   (e) Nitric oxide

   Answer: (c) Although the ureter receives neurologic input from numerous sources, spontaneous electrical activity initiated by the pacemaker cells appears to be the dominant control necessary for providing electrical activity and inducing coordinated peristaltic muscular activity. Evidence to support this contention includes the persistence of peristalsis after renal transplantation or denervation. Propagation of electrical activity proceeds through tight areas of cell-to-cell contact termed intermediate junctions.

3. All of the following statements regarding the prevention of retrograde urine flow are true with the exception of:

   (a) The ratio of intramural ureteral length/ureteral diameter plays an important role in the prevention of vesicoureteral reflux
   (b) In order for the antirefluxing mechanism to operate effectively there must exist adequate muscle backing against which the ureter can be compressed
   (c) The distal end of the ureter must be adequately anchored to the base of the

bladder so that with filling it does not migrate laterally and experience a shortening of tunnel length

(d) Maintenance of unidirectional urine flow at the ureterovesical junction (UVJ) is a purely passive process

Answer: (d)   Although the traditional concept of the ureterovesical antireflux mechanism consisted solely of a passive flap valve mechanism, a number of investigators have noted sufficient anatomic and physiological evidence to point to an active sphincteric mechanism. Although an anatomically defined circumferential sphincter has not been identified the longitudinal muscles of the UVJ are postulated to provide this "active" component by closing the meatus.

4. All of the following statements regarding ureteral physiology are true with the exception of:

(a) Under normal conditions, peristaltic contractions occur 2–6 times/min

(b) Peristaltic waves elevate ureteral pressure to 20–80 cmH$_2$O

(c) Peristaltic contractions advance down the ureters at a rate of 2–6 ml/s

(d) The ureter maintains a higher resting pressure than the bladder, thereby facilitating flow of urine in the caudal direction

Answer: (d)   The resting pressure within the ureter, 0–5 cmH$_2$O, is similar to the intravesical pressure of the nondistended bladder. Peristaltic waves elevate this pressure to 20–80 cmH$_2$O. If the intraureteral pressure exceeds the intravesical pressure urine will proceed into the bladder.

5. Which one of the following is false regarding alterations in upper urinary tract physiology secondary to obstruction?

(a) Increased luminal diameter secondary to obstruction results in an increase in intraluminal pressure

(b) Superimposed infection in the presence of obstruction can further reduce efficient peristalsis of urine

(c) Over time, the increase in urine volume held by the ureter results in decreased amplitude of peristaltic contraction waves

(d) After prolonged obstruction and the resultant deleterious effects on ureteral function, the rate of urine transport becomes dependent on hydrostatic forces generated by the kidney

Answer: (a)   As the ureter fills with urine, the peristaltic contraction waves become smaller and are unable to coapt the ureteral wall. Urine transport then becomes dependent on hydrostatic forces generated by the kidney. As predicted by the Law of Laplace, an increase in luminal size results in a decrease in intraluminal pressure, thereby decreasing the force propelling urine in a forward direction.

6. Urinary concentrating ability is the first aspect of renal function to be affected by obstruction. With increasing urine flow rates (due to the production of a larger volume of dilute urine), the initial response of the ureter is to:

(a) Increase bolus volume

(b) Increase peristaltic frequency

(c) Decrease the pressure gradient at the level of the UVJ in order to facilitate the more rapid transport of urine into the bladder

(d) Experience luminal dilation beginning at its most proximal segment

Answer: (b)   The first change in ureteral physiology resulting from an increase in urine load is to increase peristaltic frequency. After the maximal frequency is achieved, further increases in urine transport occur by means of increases in bolus volume. Eventually, the boluses coalesce and the ureter becomes filled with a continuous column of fluid.

7. Which of the following statements regarding refluxing megaureters is false?

   (a) Relative to obstructed megaureters there appears to be a higher collagen to smooth muscle ratio within the ureteral wall
   (b) Multiple infections of the refluxing ureter can result in progressive fibrosis
   (c) The collagen subtype III appears to be abnormally elevated
   (d) Surgical results are generally reported to be better in the repair of refluxing megaureters relative to obstructed megaureters

Answer: (d) Refluxing megaureters have been shown to have a twofold increase in tissue matrix ratio of collagen to smooth muscle when compared to patients with primary obstructed megaureter and controls. Investigators subsequently demonstrated that there was a greater contribution of type III collagen in the refluxing megaureter and felt that this may play a role in the pathophysiology of refluxing megaureters. Because type III collagen is a less distensible fiber, it may cause an intrinsically stiffer ureter and play a role in the lower surgical success in the reimplantation of refluxing megaureters.

8. Which of the following statements regarding the obstructed megaureter is false?

   (a) Long-standing obstruction can result in altered hierarchy of the ureteral pacemakers, resulting in cranially directed peristalsis thereby contributing to upper tract dilatation
   (b) In the primary obstructed megaureter, obstruction is due to compromise of the intravesical ureteral diameter
   (c) The Law of Laplace predicts that surgically reducing the ureteral diameter will increase intraluminal pressures
   (d) Concentrating ability is the first aspect of renal function to be affected by obstruction

Answer: (b) The classic example of a functional obstruction is the primary obstructed megaureter in which there exists an adynamic segment of distal ureter with adequate ureteral diameter. With all forms of ureteral obstruction the hierarchal order of the ureteral pacemakers may become altered. When alternate pacemakers fire, electrical activity and subsequent peristalsis can propagate both caudally and cranially from the site at which it is initiated. This lack of coordination affects the efficiency of urine transport and contributes to upper tract dilatation. The effect of ureteral diameter on the ability to generate effective peristaltic contractions provides the rationale for ureteral tapering in the patient with an increased ureteral size. The Law of Laplace would result in higher intraluminal pressures and a resultant improvement in urine transport.

9. Which statement is true regarding gender differences in regard to vesicoureteral reflux identified in the newborn?

   (a) Males are more likely to have abnormalities at the level of the UVJ that predispose to vesicoureteral reflux
   (b) Intravesical pressures are generally higher in newborn males than females, potentially explaining why newborn males tend to present with higher grades of reflux than their female cohorts
   (c) Females tend to have higher grades of reflux than males
   (d) Females have a higher genetic predisposition to develop reflux

Answer: (b) Transient urodynamic abnormalities have been identified in neurologically normal children who present with urinary tract infections (UTIs) and reflux in the first year of life. One study identified abnormalities, including detrusor hyperreflexia and elevated filling pressures, in 97% of boys and 77% of girls who presented in infancy with reflux. Intravesical pressures in boys were found to be higher than in girls, a finding confirmed by other investigators. This finding may account for gender differences in degree of reflux.

10. The most common cause(s) of secondary reflux is/are:
    (a) Posterior urethral valves
    (b) Bladder diverticuli
    (c) Ureteroceles
    (d) Bladder dysfunction

Answer: (d) The most common anatomic cause of secondary vesicoureteral reflux is posterior urethral valves, in which approximately 50% of boys are affected. However, functional causes of increased intravesical pressure, including detrusor sphincter dyssynergia in patients with neuropathic bladder dysfunction secondary to myelomeningocele, are far more common.

The imaging of reflux and ureteral disease

37

Jeanne S Chow and David A Diamond

1. A voiding cystourethrography (VCUG) is definitely preferred to a radionuclide cystogram (RNC) when studying:

   (a) Abnormalities of the male urethra
   (b) Patients with suspected duplex renal anomalies
   (c) Patients with ureteroceles
   (d) Patients with sibling reflux
   (e) Patients with cystitis

      (i) (a)
      (ii) (a) and (b)
      (iii) (a), (b) and (c)
      (iv) (a), (b), (c) and (d)
      (v) All of the above

   Answer: (iii) The VCUG enables one to precisely define the anatomy of the urethra, bladder, and ureters when reflux is present, whereas the RNC provides less anatomic detail and essentially determines the presence or absence of reflux. Therefore, to obtain anatomic definition of the male urethra, a ureterocele within the bladder or to determine that a ureter is part of the duplex system, the VCUG is required.

2. What is the initial imaging study recommended for the evaluation of the ureter?

   (a) Computerized tomography (CT)
   (b) Ultrasound
   (c) Voiding cystourethrogram
   (d) Retrograde urethrogram
   (e) Magnetic resonance imaging (MRI)

   Answer: (b) Although each of these imaging studies may be useful to evaluate the ureter, the best first imaging test would be ultrasound. Ultrasound is readily available, noninvasive, and does not emit ionizing radiation.

3. Some of the main clinical indications for ultrasound include:

   (a) Evaluation of reflux and prenatal hydronephrosis
   (b) Evaluation of stone disease and ureteral trauma
   (c) Evaluation of prenatal hydronephrosis and stone disease
   (d) Evaluation for a mid-ureteral stricture and reflux
   (e) Evaluation for stone disease and reflux

   Answer: (c) Ultrasound misses 75% of reflux. Therefore, (a), (d) and (e) would be incorrect answers. It is also a poor modality, in general, for evaluating ureteral trauma relative to a contrast study such as CT scan which can better delineate urinary extravasation.

4. MAG3 studies are useful in the evaluation of:

   (a) Reflux
   (b) Hydronephrosis
   (c) Pyelonephritis
   (d) Complex ureteral anatomy
   (e) Posterior urethral valves

   Answer: (b) MAG3 is a substance that is filtered and excreted by the kidney, and can be used to assess renal function and drainage. It is, therefore, an ideal substance with which to assess hydronephrosis. Because it does not afford precise anatomic detail it is not useful in assessing complex ureteral anatomy.

5. The main disadvantage of MR urography compared to other imaging studies is:

   (a) Long imaging time often requiring sedation
   (b) Difficulty imaging patients with poor renal function
   (c) Difficulty in imaging infants with "renal immaturity"
   (d) Inadequate visualization of the ureters
   (e) Poor contrast resolution

   Answer: (a) MR urography affords precise definition of ureteral anatomy and is not dependent upon renal function. However, it does require a long imaging time (30–45 min). For young or uncooperative children this is likely to require sedation.

Ureteral anomalies and their surgical management

38

Christopher Cooper

1. Which of the following mid-ureteral surgical techniques is most likely to result in ureteral stricture?

   (a) Renal mobilization
   (b) Ureteral stents
   (c) Removal of periureteral adventitia
   (d) Peri-anastomotic drains
   (e) Spatulation of both proximal and distal ureteral segments

   Answer: (c) The blood supply to the mid-ureter is more tenuous than that of the proximal and distal ureter. The adventitia supports multiple blood vessels, and to preserve the adventitia and blood supply the ureter should be mobilized with as much surrounding soft tissue as possible. Removal of the adventitial layer may result in ischemic injury and subsequent ureteral stricture. Renal mobilization, drainage, and spatulation are all techniques which may be employed to result in a tension-free wide-open anastomosis.

2. A retrocaval ureter is most often associated with which of the following:

   (a) Persistence of the supracardinal vein
   (b) The left ureter
   (c) Hematuria
   (d) Lateral ureteral displacement
   (e) Absence of symptoms

   Answer: (e) Most patients with a retrocaval ureter are asymptomatic, but some present with obstructive symptoms. The retrocaval ureter is almost always on the right and is displaced medially most often at the L3 level. The persistence of the *sub*cardinal vein results in the development of the retrocaval ureter.

3. A 14-year-old child presents with intermittent left flank pain and gross hematuria. Intravenous pyelogram (IVP) reveals a long, smooth-filling defect in the distal ureter. Cystoscopy reveals a polypoid lesion projecting from the ureteral orifice and biopsy reveals epithelial-lined fibrovascular fronds. Appropriate treatment may require:

   (a) Nephrectomy
   (b) Nephroureterectomy
   (c) Transurethral resection and Bacille Calmette-Guérin (BCG)
   (d) Upper tract instillation of BCG
   (e) None of the above

   Answer: (e) This patient has a benign fibroepithelial polyp. Appropriate treatment is by complete resection. This may be approached by ureteroscopy from the bladder or percutaneously from the kidney. At times, ureterotomy may be required to completely remove the polyp and the base of its stalk.

Megaureter

39

Douglass Clayton

1. The ureter receives its blood supply predominately from:

   (a) Renal artery
   (b) Aorta
   (c) Internal iliac artery
   (d) Gonadal artery
   (e) All of the above

   Answer: (e)   The blood supply of the ureter is not based solely on one vessel, instead it is supplied by multiple branches from various arteries. The blood flow to the proximal ureter originates in the ipsilateral renal artery while the mid-ureter receives its blood supply both from direct aortic branches and from branches of the gonadal artery. Finally, the distal ureteral blood supply arises from the internal iliac artery as well as the superior and inferior vesical arteries. All of these various sources of blood supply then form an anastomotic network of vessels that travels within the adventitia of the ureter.

2. Megaureter is defined as having a ureteral diameter greater than:

   (a) 4 mm
   (b) 5 mm
   (c) 6 mm
   (d) 7 mm
   (e) 8 mm

   Answer: (e)   Studies of ureteral diameter in children involving both postmortem analysis and excretory urography analysis have shown the normal diameter of the pediatric ureter is <6 mm in size. Thus, the accepted definition for megaureter is a ureter >8 mm in diameter.

3. Patients with refluxing megaureter are found to have an increase in which of the following types of collagen fibers:

   (a) Type I
   (b) Type II
   (c) Type III
   (d) Type IV

   Answer: (c)   Previous authors have shown a relative increase in the presence of Type I and Type III collagen both in the obstructed megaureter as well as the refluxing megaureter. However, in the refluxing megaureter, the proportion of Type III collagen is increased predominately and may result in a ureter which is less distensible than other megaureter types.

4. A diagnosis of megaureter is identified in approximately how many asymptomatic neonates:

   (a) 5%
   (b) 10%
   (c) 25%
   (d) 50%
   (e) 75%

   Answer: (c)   Approximately 25% of neonates are found to have megaureter on routine fetal sonography. The only entity more commonly noted is that of hydronephrosis which is identified in up to 41% of fetal ultrasounds.

5. When evaluating the function of the megaureter, the diagnostic study which provides the greatest amount of data is:

   (a) Ultrasonography
   (b) Renal scintigraphy

(c) Magnetic resonance urography

(d) Whitaker test

(e) Voiding cystourethrography (VCUG)

Answer: (b) Of the studies mentioned above, renal scintigraphy is the only study which provides adequate functional data. Both ultrasonography and VCUG are necessary components of the evaluation of megaureter. Ultrasound provides good anatomic data of both ureter and the kidney. Likewise, the VCUG characterizes the anatomy of the lower urinary tract and is essential in evaluating for vesicoureteral reflux. Magnetic resonance urography is a burgeoning test and may provide improved anatomic detail. The Whitaker test is invasive and is not routinely performed today.

6. The radiotracer of choice when performing neonatal renal scintigraphy for the evaluation of the megaureter is:

(a) DMSA

(b) DTPA

(c) MAG3

Answer: (c) Because of the immature state of the neonatal renal unit when renal scintigraphy is performed with radiotracers which approximate glomerular filtration rate such as DTPA, limited data are provided regarding the degree of ureteral obstruction. Of the available agents for neonatal scintigraphy, mercaptoacetyltriglycine (MAG3) is the agent of choice because it provides functional data based on the effective renal plasma flow of the kidney not the neonatal glomerular filtration rate.

7. The procedure of choice for temporary urinary diversion in the patient with obstructed megaureter is:

(a) Percutaneous nephrostomy

(b) Cutaneous ureterostomy

(c) Vesicostomy

(d) Pyelostomy

Answer: (b) A subset of patients with obstructed megaureter and renal impairment may benefit from temporary urinary diversion. Diversion may allow for decompression of the ureter, resolution of infection, and improvement in renal function. Of the available diversion procedures, cutaneous ureterostomy is the procedure of choice due to its low morbidity and effectiveness.

8. Definitive reconstruction of the megaureter is best undertaken when the child is:

(a) Newborn

(b) 6 months of age

(c) 8 months of age

(d) 12 months of age

(e) 24 months of age

Answer: (d) The technical difficulties of surgical correction of the megaureter are less when performed after 12 months of age. Previous studies have demonstrated that as many as 10% of infants undergoing reconstruction at <8 months of age will require repeat procedures.

9. The principles of surgery for the megaureter include which of the following:

(a) Adequate straightening of the ureter

(b) Tapering without devascularization

(c) 5:1 ureteral tunnel to diameter length

(d) Antirefluxing repair

(e) All of the above

Answer: (e) All of the principles listed above should be considered when repair of the megaureter is undertaken. Extensive ureteral dissection may result in devascularization of the ureteral segment. Tapering should be limited to the intramural portion of the ureter only. A gradual transition should occur from the tapered to nontapered segment to decrease the risk of a pseudo-obstruction.

10. Persistent vesicoureteral reflux after tapered reimplant for megaureter occurs in what percentage of patients:

(a) 5%
(b) 15%
(c) 20%
(d) 30%
(e) 50%

Answer: (a)   After a tapered ureteral reimplant, a voiding cystourethrogram should be performed at 6 months. Once the absence of reflux is confirmed, any antibiotic prophylaxis may be discontinued. Up to 5% of patients will have persistent reflux after a tapered reimplant. This should be monitored initially as many will resolve within a few months of surgery. Those patients with continued reflux may require a repeat procedure.

Ureteral duplication anomalies: ectopic ureters and ureteroceles

40

Jorge R Caso and Michael A Keating

1. Which of the following statements about ureteral development is false?

   (a) Wolffian duct remnants in the female include Gartner's duct, the epoophoron and oophoron; an ectopic ureter venting into these bypasses the external sphincter, causing incontinence

   (b) An ectopic ureter in a male will drain into structures proximal to the urinary sphincter, such as the seminal vesicle, vas deferens, or prostatic urethra

   (c) If the ureteral bud originates from a more cephalad than usual position on the mesonephric duct, primary reflux from the resultant short submucosal ureter can occur

   (d) After the common excretory duct is absorbed into the bladder and the ureteral orifice begins its migration, the excretory duct continues moving toward the midline, fusing to its contralateral partner to form the primitive trigone

   (e) In a duplicated kidney, the superior/upper pole ureteric bud may assume an abnormally high position along the mesonephric duct, while the lower pole bud may be positioned more caudally than usual; the resultant relationship of ureteral orifice to draining renal segment is defined by the Weigert-Meyer law

   Answer: (c)   After the ureteral orifice is absorbed into the bladder it migrates in a cranial and lateral direction. A more caudally positioned ureteral bud will be absorbed into the bladder more quickly, migrate a greater distance, and become more laterally exaggerated. Vesicoureteral reflux can result.

2. Which of the following statements about ureteroceles is false?

   (a) Theories about the origins of ureteroceles include: persistence of Chwalla's membrane; abnormal muscular development of the terminal ureter, possibly in conjunction with meatal or perisphincteric obstruction; and abnormal widening of the mesonephric duct between its insertion in the urogenital sinus and the ureteral bud

   (b) Ureteroceles commonly cause unilateral hydronephrosis from ureteral blockage

   (c) Salvageable renal function is usually seen with extravesical ureteroceles, while intravesical ureteroceles are associated with poor function

   (d) Ureteroceles occur more frequently than ectopic ureters (1:500 versus 1:2000), are more common in females, and are associated with duplex systems in females 95% of the time whereas in 66% of males there is a single system

   Answer: (c)   Intravesical ureteroceles are more commonly associated with salvageable renal function and extravesical ureteroceles with poor function. This may be explained by an abnormal takeoff of the ureteral bud inducing less favorable polar tissue of the metanephric blastema to develop. Cystic dysplasia could result.

3. Which of the following statements about the classification of ureteroceles is false?

    (a) According to Stephens' classification, intravesical ureteroceles are either stenotic or nonobstructed, while extravesical ureteroceles are classified as sphincteric, sphincterostenotic, cecoureteroceles, or blind ectopic

    (b) Intravesical stenotic and extravesical sphincteric ureteroceles are the most common variants

    (c) Sphincteric ureteroceles always open proximal to the sphincter

    (d) Cecoureteroceles open into the bladder, but have a blind pouch extending into the submucosa of the urethra which may cause bladder outlet obstruction when distended with urine

    (e) Blind ectopic ureteroceles are similar to the sphincteric variants, but without a ureteral orifice

    Answer: (c)   Generally, sphincteric ureteroceles open proximal to the external sphincter. However, in females the meatus is sometimes distally positioned. At rest, the bladder neck and sphincter contract, which can obstruct the ureter and orifice.

4. All of the following statements about the presentation of ureteroceles and ectopic ureters are true except:

    (a) Prolapsed ureteroceles have a pink, smooth wall, unlike the grape-like appearance of sarcoma botryoides or the yellow-white color of a periurethral duct cyst

    (b) Ureteroceles typically present with a urinary tract infection (UTI), failure to thrive, and colic; ectopic ureters commonly present with flank pain, fever, and an abdominal mass

    (c) The diagnosis of ureteral ectopia should be entertained in any girl who reportedly has never been fully toilet trained

    (d) In males, ectopic ureters may cause prostatitis, seminal vesiculitis, and epididymitis

    (e) An extravesical ureterocele is the most common cause of bladder outlet obstruction in newborn girls and boys

    Answer: (e)   Posterior urethral valves are the most common cause of bladder outlet obstruction in newborn boys; an extravesical ureterocele is the second most common cause.

5. All of the following statements about the radiographic appearance of ureteroceles and ectopic ureters are true except:

    (a) Ectopic ureters that displace the bladder can often be differentiated from ureteroceles by noting the thickness of the wall that separates the structure from the bladder lumen

    (b) Radionuclide scans in the newborn that are completed soon after delivery offer the most accurate assessment of renal function with both anomalies

    (c) Vesicoureteral reflux occurs in the ipsilateral lower pole moiety with both ureteroceles and ectopic ureters about 50% of the time

    (d) Excretory urography is especially useful in the diagnosis of ectopic ureters and may be suggestive of nonfunctioning, occult duplications

    Answer: (b)   The transitional physiology of the newborn kidney affects its handling of radionuclides and contrast. Function can be underestimated and later recovery overestimated if scans are completed during the first few days of life. Radionuclide studies should be deferred for at least 4–6 weeks.

6. Which of the following statements regarding the management of ectopic ureters is false?

    (a) After performing nephrectomy for an ectopic ureter associated with a minimally functioning kidney, a nonrefluxing, obstructed ureteral stump should be left open to drain

(b) For a duplex system with marginally functioning upper pole, when considering salvage and evaluating relative function, one should note that the upper pole moiety provides about one-third of the affected kidney's function in a normal duplex kidney

(c) In a single system anomaly having salvageable function, reimplantation should be carried out disregarding the distal-most ureteral segment entering the urethra or bladder neck

(d) In a duplex system having salvageable function, ureteropyelostomy (the lower pole renal pelvis) or ureteroureterostomy are recommended treatments.

Answer: (a) When a ureteral stump is left, it should be taken as distally as possible, ligated with absorbable sutures, and urine aspirated from its distal end. Reflux can be associated with obstructed ectopic ureters but can be unappreciated unless cyclic voiding cystourethrography is included in the work-up. In such cases a urinary fistula can develop if the stump is left open.

7. Which of the following treatments regarding the management of ureteroceles is false?

(a) With single system ureteroceles, nephrectomy is the treatment of choice for those associated with minimal or nonfunctioning kidneys

(b) Upper pole heminephrectomy is recommended for duplex systems having minimally or nonfunctioning upper poles; however, lower urinary reconstruction is still required of a significant (20–30%) number of patients

(c) In a single system associated with a salvageable kidney, selective incision and puncture is the procedure of choice

(d) In a duplex system having a functioning upper pole, the majority of patients will require surgery of the upper and lower urinary tracts when vesicoureteral reflux is present in two or more associated renal moieties

Answer: (d) The majority of these patients, especially older children, can be managed solely at the bladder level, excising the ureterocele and correcting the reflux, thus eliminating the need for secondary surgery.

8. Which of the following is not recommended when performing cystoscopic incision of a ureterocele?

(a) Aggressive hydration and minimal use of intravesical irrigation are helpful for keeping the ureterocele distended

(b) The puncture can be performed with a fine Bugbee electrode using cutting current; a laser can also be used

(c) Selective punctures of intravesical ureteroceles are created along their lateral edge

(d) Follow-up includes an ultrasound 10–14 days later to document resolution of hydronephrosis and decompression of the ureterocele

(e) A voiding cystourethrogram should be performed 3–6 months later in evaluation of reflux

Answer: (c) Selective incisions are placed at a distal position along the medial base of the ureterocele. The intent is to preserve enough submucosal length to obviate the development of reflux. With cecoureteroceles and sphincteric ureteroceles, the meatus should be incised vertically and the cut extended above the bladder neck.

9. Which of the following statements regarding surgical technique is false?

(a) Traction should be minimized in all patients when mobilizing the kidney, but especially in babies, who are prone to vascular spasm and intimal tears; papaverine can be applied topically if vascular spasm persists

(b) Heminephrectomy defects should be closed with chromic mattress sutures incorporating the parenchyma and fascia; pararenal fat may also be mobilized and tacked into position to close the defect

(c) After performing a heminephrectomy, tacking the capsule of the lower pole of the kidney to muscle is recommended to avoid postoperative torsion

(d) When performing a lower ureterectomy, the ureter can be identified by ligating the obliterated hypogastric artery and following it laterally until the ureter is encountered posteriorly

Answer: (d) Once the hypogastric artery is identified, it should be followed posteriorly until the ureter is encountered medially.

10. Which of the following statements regarding the postoperative management of ureterocele surgery is false?

(a) When bladder reconstruction becomes necessary after incision of a ureterocele in a newborn, it is reasonable to address the problem at about 1 year of age

(b) Addressing ureteroceles at an age prior to toilet training is optimal because children who are corrected at an early age rarely develop bladder dysfunction

(c) If vesicoureteral reflux is noted on the initial follow-up cystogram after ureterocele repair, a trial of medical management is reasonable; however, the rate of spontaneous resolution is less than that encountered with primary reflux

(d) In general, prophylactic antibiotics should be continued after surgery until postoperative studies confirm the adequacy of the repair

(e) After the anomaly has been corrected, a reasonable follow-up would include ultrasound studies at 2 and 5 years, as well as exams by the primary physicians to include checking urine, blood pressure, and interval somatic growth

Answer: (b) Bladder dysfunction is quite common after surgical repair even when performed prior to toilet training (up to two-thirds of children). Infrequent voiding, large capacities, and significant post-void residuals are typical findings.

Laparoscopic management of duplication anomalies

41

Stephen Lukasewycz and Aseem R Shukla

(Based on chapter written by Alberto Lais and Craig Peters)

1. What are the technical advantages of a retroperitoneal versus a transperitoneal approach to laparoscopic management of duplication anomalies?

    (a) A retroperitoneal approach offers wider field of view
    (b) A retroperitoneal approach allows for easy access to other genitourinary structures allowing for concomitant surgery (i.e. orchiopexy)
    (c) A retroperitoneal approach allows for a larger working space and therefore larger insufflation volumes
    (d) A retroperitoneal approach allows essentially direct access to the renal unit and minimizes the risk of postoperative adhesions secondary to bowel mobilization
    (e) A retroperioneal approach results in a significantly shorter operative time

    Answer: (d) Owing to the size of the peritoneum compared to the retroperitoneal space created by insufflation, a transperitoneal approach allows for a wider field of view and a larger working space. Additionally, a transperitoneal approach allows for easier access to other genitourinary structures compared to a retroperitoneal approach. Recent studies have failed to show a difference in operative time in a transperitoneal versus a retroperitoneal approach. A retroperitoneal approach does offer essentially direct access to the renal unit and, as the peritoneum is not entered, limits the risk of future adhesions.

2. All of the following are true when comparing a laparoscopic partial nephrectomy and an open approach in the pediatric population except:

    (a) Shorter operative time
    (b) Shorter hospital stay
    (c) Decreased need for postoperative analgesia
    (d) High rate of conversion of laparoscopic procedure to open procedure
    (e) None of the above

    Answer: (a) At some centers with a large laparoscopic experience, laparoscopic surgery often allows for a shorter hospital stay and a decreased need for postoperative analgesia; however, operative times are generally equivalent or longer compared to open surgery. The rate of conversion to an open procedure is very low in most series.

3. If during a laparoscopic upper pole partial nephrectomy, the lower pole remnant begins to appear blue and ischemic, one should:

    (a) Perform lower pole nephrectomy
    (b) Release all tension off the lower pole vessels
    (c) Apply neosynephrine directly to the lower pole vessels
    (d) Decrease pneumoperitoneum pressure
    (e) (b) and (c)

    Answer: (b) During laparoscopic partial nephrectomy, manipulation of the lower pole moiety may lead to arterial vasospasm and decreased blood flow. Releasing tension on the lower pole vessels and applying papaverine or lidocaine directly to the affected vessels may reverse this condition.

4. All of the following are true for robotic laparoscopy as compared to traditional laparoscopy in pediatric urologic surgery except:

   (a) Improved visualization with high definition and three-dimensional capabilities
   (b) Increased speed and easier fine suturing capabilities
   (c) Increased field of surgery due to versatility and mobility of robot
   (d) Lack of tactile feedback requiring reliance on visual cues
   (e) None of the above

Answer: (c)   A limitation of robotic laparoscopy is that once the robot is engaged, no further adjustment to patient position is possible without disengaging the robot and resetting the arms into newly placed ports. Robotic laparoscopy also lacks tactile feedback, and the surgeon must rely on the appearance of tissue during grasping and an understanding of the inherent strength of the robotic arm when manipulating intraabdominal structures.

Vesicoureteral reflux: anatomic and functional basis of etiology

42

John M Park

1. Which of the following statements is *not* true of the normal ureterovesical junction (UVJ) anatomy and function?

   (a) The inner longitudinal muscle fibers of the ureter extend into the superficial trigone
   (b) Waldeyer's sheath anchors the intramural ureter and prevents displacement during bladder filling
   (c) Contraction of the trigonal musculature causes lateral displacement of the ureteric orifice
   (d) Embryologically, both ureter and trigone develop from mesonephric duct origin

   Answer: (c)   Contraction of the trigonal musculature anchors the ureter and prevents the lateral displacement of the ureteric orifice. All other statements are true.

2. The "flap-valve" mechanism of the UVJ is reinforced by the following *except*:

   (a) An adequate length of the intramural ureter and submucosal tunnel
   (b) Sturdy back wall support of the detrusor muscle
   (c) Well-integrated ureter-trigone muscle complex
   (d) Paraureteral diverticulum

   Answer: (d)   Paraureteral diverticulum lacks an adequate detrusor muscle support and causes the intramural ureter to displace extravesically during bladder filling. Consequently, there is a shortening of the intramural ureter and a loss of flap-valve mechanism.

3. Which of the following demographic statements is *true* of vesicoureteral reflux (VUR)?

   (a) In infancy, VUR is more common and of severe grade in girls
   (b) VUR is most common in patients with Asian ancestry
   (c) The incidence of VUR in normal infants and children is estimated to be 0.4–1.8%, whereas in children with UTI it can be up to 30–50%
   (d) In familial analysis, VUR does not appear to be a heritable disorder

   Answer: (c)   In infants, VUR is more common and of severe grade in boys. VUR is most commonly found in patients with Caucasian racial background and is rare in those of Asian and African ancestry. There is an increased incidence of VUR among siblings as well as children of patients with VUR, indicating its heritable nature.

4. The most commonly found voiding dysfunction in older girls with VUR is:

   (a) Detrusor instability with detrusor sphincter dyssynergia
   (b) Detrusor areflexia
   (c) High-pressure voiding
   (d) High postvoid residual

   Answer: (a)   Detrusor areflexia is possible but uncommon. High-pressure voiding is most frequently seen in infant boys with VUR. High postvoid residual can be seen but is not the most common voiding dysfunction.

5. The appropriate clinical management of VUR in children must include consideration of:

   (a) Anatomic UVJ competency
   (b) Potential bladder dysfunction
   (c) Predisposition to urinary tract infection (UTI)
   (d) Underlying renal dysplasia
   (e) All of the above

   Answer: (e)   The distinction between *primary* and *secondary* VUR is important in the conceptualization of contributing pathophysiology and relevant anatomic/functional etiologies which need to be addressed clinically. In all patients presenting with VUR, the proper management must include a global view of the entire urinary tract, including UVJ mechanism, bladder dysfunction, predisposition to UTI, and renal anomalies.

6. The *secondary* VUR may be caused by the following entities *except*:

   (a) Posterior urethral valves
   (b) Neurogenic bladder dysfunction
   (c) Non-neurogenic bladder dysfunction
   (d) Primary nocturnal enuresis

   Answer: (d)   *Primary* VUR is thought to represent an abnormal anatomy and function of the UVJ, whereas *secondary* VUR implies an acquired condition as a result of increased intravesical pressure in the setting of neurogenic bladder dysfunction, non-neurogenic bladder dysfunction, or outlet obstruction.

Nonsurgical management of vesicoureteral reflux

43

Jack S Elder

1. A 4-year-old girl with left grade III vesicoureteral reflux (VUR) develops a urinary tract infection (UTI) with left flank pain and a temperature of 103°F. A DMSA scan shows acute pyelonephritis:

   (a) In <5% of cases
   (b) In 15–20% of cases
   (c) In 40–50% of cases
   (d) Most often in the presence of voiding dysfunction
   (e) Only if treatment is delayed for 4–7 days

   Answer: (b)   Children with reflux who are receiving antibiotic prophylaxis are at risk for acute pyelonephritis. According to Szlyk et al, the risk is 17%, irrespective of age, gender, and presence of preexisting renal scarring.[1]

2. In the dysfunctional voiding scoring system (DVSS), which of the following is not included:

   (a) When I pee it hurts
   (b) I wet the bed at night
   (c) I have to push to pee
   (d) When I wee myself, my underwear is soaked
   (e) I only go to the bathroom one or two times per day

   Answer: (b)   The DVSS includes ten items pertaining to voiding and bowel habits; seven items pertain to bladder function, two pertain to bowel function, and one pertains to a stressful event related to their voiding pattern. Each item is scored from 0 to 3; 0 is almost never, 1 is less than half the time, 2 is about half the time, and 3 is almost every time. A higher score is indicative of more severe voiding dysfunction.[2]

3. In the DVSS which of the following components yields a low score:

   (a) Flow rate >18 ml/s
   (b) Postvoid residual urine volume <10% predicted maximum bladder volume
   (c) Absence of uninhibited bladder contractions on urodynamic studies
   (d) Bowel movement once per day
   (e) Reflux grade II or less

   Answer: (d)   The DVSS includes ten items pertaining to voiding and bowel habits; seven items pertain to bladder function, two pertain to bowel function, and one pertains to a stressful event related to their voiding pattern. Each item is scored from 0 to 3; 0 is almost never, 1 is less than half the time, 2 is about half the time, and 3 is almost every time. A higher score is indicative of more severe voiding dysfunction. It does not include urodynamic data.[2]

4. When administered before a voiding cystourethrography (VCUG), oral midazolam often causes:

   (a) Anterograde amnesia
   (b) Sedation

(c) Oxygen desaturation

(d) Hypotension

(e) Impaired voiding

Answer: (a)   Oral midazolam causes anxiolysis and anterograde amnesia, but not significant sedation. Although children are monitored, changes in oxygen saturation or vital signs are uncommon. It does not inhibit voiding to any significant degree. Unlike propofol, it does not cause significant sedation.[3]

5. A 5-year-old girl develops a febrile UTI. The renal sonogram is normal. A VCUG shows bilateral grade II VUR. If medical management is recommended, 2 years after diagnosis, the risk of persistent reflux is approximately:

(a) 20%

(b) 40%

(c) 60%

(d) 80%

(e) Higher than if there was only unilateral reflux

Answer: (c)   According to the data generated by the AUA Pediatric Reflux Guidelines panel, in grade I and II VUR, the spontaneous resolution rate is similar for unilateral and bilateral reflux, and does not vary with age. With grade II reflux, 80% show reflux resolution at 5 years. The likelihood of spontaneous resolution is fairly constant each year, although in the first few years the resolution rate is slightly higher.[4]

6. A 2-year-old girl develops a febrile urinary tract infection. A DMSA scan shows renal scarring in the left kidney. A VCUG demonstrates grade III VUR on the right and grade IV VUR on the right. If long-term medical management is chosen, the likelihood of persistent reflux at 10 years is approximately:

(a) 20%

(b) 40%

(c) 60%

(d) 80%

(e) Nearly 100%

Answer: (c)   In the International Reflux Study, at 5 years, only 10% of children with grade III–IV reflux randomized to medical therapy showed spontaneous resolution. However, at 10 years, 39% had shown spontaneous resolution. In contrast, with unilateral grade III–IV VUR, 73% had shown spontaneous resolution, and in children with grade III–IV on one side and grade I–II on the other, 49% had resolved.[5]

7. In children, compared with sulfamethoxazole-trimethoprim, which of the following side-effects of nitrofurantoin is more common:

(a) Stevens-Johnson syndrome

(b) Hives

(c) Photosensitivity

(d) Hepatotoxicity

(e) Hemolytic anemia

Answer: (e)   Photosensitivity and delayed allergic reaction are the most common side-effects associated with treatment with sulfamethoxazole-trimethoprim. Other less common side-effects include leucopenia, hepatotoxicity, and, in rare cases, Stevens-Johnson syndrome. Side-effects with nitrofurantoin also are common and include hepatotoxicity, cutaneous reaction, pulmonary fibrosis, and hemolytic anemia in patients who have glucose-6-phosphate dehydrogenase deficiency. Nausea is far more common with the nitrofurantoin suspension, but less common with macrocrystals.[6]

8. In children with an overactive bladder, treatment with anticholinergic medication is associated with all of the following except:

(a) Xerostomia

(b) Blurred vision

(c) Higher resolution rate of VUR

(d) Diarrhea

(e) Drowsiness

Answer: (d) Typical side-effects of anticholinergics include xerostomia (dry mouth), facial flushing, reduced sweating, constipation, and less commonly, blurred vision and drowsiness. Side-effects are dose related and may be eliminated with dose reduction. Alteration in mental function has not been observed.

9. In children with dysfunctional voiding and VUR, biofeedback therapy:

   (a) Should be supplemented with anticholinergic therapy
   (b) Is associated with increased likelihood of reflux resolution
   (c) Should be supplemented with laxative therapy
   (d) Should not be used if the postvoid residual urine volume is >15% of the child's expected bladder capacity
   (e) Is usually unsuccessful in children with day and night incontinence

Answer: (b) In children with dysfunctional voiding, typically there is inconsistent relaxation of the external sphincter during voiding. This pattern may occur because of an overactive bladder which causes the child to tighten his or her sphincter during a detrusor contraction. A typical treatment session might include a uroflow study, sonographic evaluation of postvoid residual urine volume, and a 1 h session with perineal patch electrodes for electromyography. Often, this treatment is used instead of anticholinergic therapy or in children who fail that treatment. However, some children need supplemental anticholinergic therapy. In addition, in children with significant constipation, oral laxative therapy is important. It is associated with an increased likelihood of reflux resolution.[7]

10. According to the AUA Practice Guidelines report, in a child with reflux diagnosed following a UTI, which of the following is associated with the highest likelihood of spontaneous reflux resolution?

    (a) Unilateral grade III VUR, diagnosed at 4 years of age
    (b) Unilateral grade IV VUR, diagnosed at 2 years of age
    (c) Bilateral grade II VUR, diagnosed at 6 years of age
    (d) Bilateral grade III VUR, diagnosed at 1 year of age
    (e) Bilateral grade IV VUR, diagnosed at 1 year of age

Answer: (c) According to the AUA Practice Guidelines, reflux resolution for grades I and II VUR is independent of the age of the patient and laterality (unilateral versus bilateral). In contrast, with grade III VUR, the likelihood of reflux resolution is lower with higher age at diagnosis and for bilateral versus unilateral VUR. For grade IV VUR there are insufficient patient numbers to draw any conclusions regarding age at diagnosis and laterality. At 5 years, the likelihood of reflux resolution for unilateral grade III VUR diagnosed at 4 years of age is 50%, for unilateral grade IV VUR diagnosed at 2 years of age is 50%, for bilateral grade II VUR diagnosed at any age is 80%, for bilateral grade III VUR diagnosed at 1 year of age is 60%, and for bilateral grade IV VUR diagnosed at any age is 10%.[4]

References

1. Szlyk GR, Williams SB, Majd M, Belman AB, Rushton HG. Incidence of new renal parenchymal inflammatory changes following breakthough urinary tract infection in patients with vesicoureteral reflux treated with antibiotic prophylaxis: evaluation by ^{99M}Technetium dimercapto-succinic acid renal scan. J Urol 2003; 170: 1566–8.
2. Farhat W, Bagli DJ, Capolicchio G et al. The dysfunctional voiding scoring system: quantitative standardization

of dysfunctional voiding symptoms in children. J Urol 2000; 164: 1011–15.

3. Elder JS, Longenecker R. Premedication with oral midazolam for voiding cystourethrography in children: safety and efficacy. Am J Roentgenol 1995; 164: 1229–332.

4. Elder JS, Peters CA, Arant BS Jr et al. Pediatric Vesicoureteral Reflux Panel Guidelines summary report on the management of vesicoureteral reflux in children. J Urol 1997; 157: 1846–51.

5. Smellie JM, Jodal U, Lax H et al. Outcome at 10 years of severe vesicoureteric reflux managed medically: report of the International Reflux Study in Children. J Pediatr 2001; 139: 656–63.

6. Karpman E, Kurzrock EA. Adverse reactions of nitrofurantoin, trimethoprim, and sulfamethoxazole in children. J Urol 2004; 172: 448–53.

7. Palmer LS, Franco I, Rotario P et al. Biofeedback therapy expedites the resolution of reflux in older children. J Urol 2002; 168: 1699–702.

Surgery for vesicoureteral reflux 44

John W Brock III and Romano T DeMarco

1. Which of the following statements regarding the surgical correction of vesicoureteral reflux (VUR) is correct?

   (a) All patients require an indwelling urethral catheter following surgery
   (b) Endoscopic subureteric injection is the current surgical "gold standard" for treatment
   (c) Persistent ureteral obstruction is common following surgical correction
   (d) New contralateral VUR following unilateral neocystostomy typically requires surgical correction
   (e) Open surgery has a 95% or greater success rate

   Answer: (e)   Open ureteral reimplantation surgery is highly successful, with reported success rates of ≥95% independent of technique. While newer, less invasive, and novel alternatives to antireflux surgery exist, open surgical repair of VUR is the only technique with a well-documented durable response. Routine urethral catheterization after surgery is not required, and may prolong convalescence and delay anticipated discharge in some patients. Ureteral obstruction has been reported to occur in about 1% of patients after surgery. New-onset contralateral reflux is typically low grade and usually resolves spontaneously with good voiding habits.

2. The modified Politano-Leadbetter repair:

   (a) Involves laparoscopic mobilization of the ureter
   (b) Was originally described 10 years ago
   (c) Was described to decrease complications related to the original procedure

   (d) Can be performed extravesically
   (e) Is only performed in children with nondilating reflux

   Answer: (c)   The original Politano-Leadbetter technique described in 1958 involved the intravesical blind creation of a new suprahiatal muscular location for the ureter. Modifications of Politano and Leadbetter's original description were made to lengthen the submucosal ureteral tunnel and prevent inadvertent injury to adjacent structures during the transfer of the ureter to its new suprahiatal location. This versatile technique is successfully used to correct all grades of reflux.

3. The major drawback related to the cross-trigonal repair described by Cohen is?

   (a) The high rate of postoperative VUR
   (b) The extensive ureteral mobilization required in this technique leading to devascularization of the ureter
   (c) The difficult intubation of the ureteral orifices encountered following surgery
   (d) The substantial risk of postoperative urinary retention
   (e) The inability to create an adequate intravesical tunnel

   Answer: (c)   The cross-trigonal repair described by Cohen is arguably today's most popular open technique for ureteral reimplantation. The success rate using this approach is close to 99% in those without dilating reflux. This method requires less ureteral mobilization than the Politano-Leadbetter repair, as the submucosal tunnel is created along the posterior bladder wall without transferring the ureter to a new muscular hiatus, virtually eliminating kinking of the distal ureter. The major drawback to this operation is the subsequent difficult intubation of the ureteral orifices related to their transtrigonal location. Transient postoperative urinary retention is occasionally encountered in children following bilateral extravesical ureteral reimplantation.

4. The Glenn-Anderson repair:

    (a) Is well suited for those patients with laterally displaced ureters
    (b) Is similar to the transtrigonal technique
    (c) Can be performed in an intra- or extravesical fashion
    (d) Has a high failure rate
    (e) Was the first method described to correct VUR

    Answer: (a) The Glenn-Anderson intravesical ureteral advancement technique is highly successful in the select patient with reflux. Those patients with laterally displaced ureters and a sufficient posterior bladder wall are ideal candidates for this advancement procedure and success rates in these properly selected patients rival other open techniques.

5. Which of the following statements is correct?

    (a) The Lich-Gregoir technique was initially described by two Russian surgeons

    (b) The Gil-Vernet advancement repair is a good option for any patient with VUR
    (c) Routine voiding cystourethrography (VCUG) is routinely performed in all patients following reimplant surgery
    (d) Open surgery is not as durable a repair as endoscopic subureteric injection for the treatment of VUR
    (e) Patients following bilateral extravesical ureteral reimplantation are at risk for developing postoperative urinary retention

    Answer: (e) An extravesical approach to the correction of VUR was almost simultaneously described in the USA and in Europe in the early 1960s. Following bilateral extravesical reimplantation, transient postoperative bladder retention has been reported and a voiding trial prior to discharge is recommended. A simple advancement technique for those patients with lateral ectopia and a widened "megatrigone" was described by Gil-Vernet in 1984 and is used in very select patients with reflux. Because of the high rate of success following open ureteral reimplantation surgery, routine postoperative voiding studies are not necessary when the surgery is performed by an experienced surgeon. In contrast to ureteroneocystostomy, questions with regard to the durability of endoscopic subureteric injection persist.

Injection therapy for vesicoureteral reflux

46

Michael A Poch and Anthony A Caldamone

1. Proper technique of injection therapy includes all of the following *except*:

   (a) Bladder distended to ¾ capacity
   (b) Needle bevel up at the 6 o'clock position
   (c) Monitor for bulging after initially injecting 1–2 ml
   (d) The use of multiple injection sites

   Answer: (d) Proper technique for the standard subureteric transurethral injection (STING) therapy involves the following steps: (1) emptying the bladder to ¾ capacity so as not to displace the ureter laterally; (2) placement of the needle bevel up into the posterior portion of the ureter; (3) visualization of the creation of the mound with initial injection of 0.1–0.2 ml of material. Multiple injection sites implies there was difficulty in obtaining a proper mound in the correct plane, as well as increasing the possibility of leakage of injectable material. Kirsch et al reported improved results by modifying the standard technique by performing hydrodistention of the ureteral orifice and injection into the submucosa of the ureteral tunnel.[1]

2. Which of the following injectable materials requires preinjection skin testing:

   (a) Polytetrafluoroethylene (PTFE)
   (b) Dextranomer/hyaluronic acid
   (c) Cross-linked bovine collagen
   (d) Polymethysiloxane

   Answer: (c) Preinjection skin testing is necessary for the use of cross-linked bovine collagen as 3% of patients will have a hypersensitivity reaction. However, a negative result does not completely eliminate the risk of an allergic reaction. Leonard et al describe a small subset of patients who developed antibovine collagen antibodies who had negative preinjection skin testing. While those patients became seropositive the clinical relevance is unclear. In only one of those patients a local reaction occurred which may have been immunogenic.[2]

3. The mechanism of long-term sustained efficacy of dextranomer/hyaluronic acid is:

   (a) Giant cell reaction and granuloma formation
   (b) Fibrous encapsulation
   (c) Fibroblast migration and collagen ingrowth
   (d) Rapid absorption and replacement with calcium carbonate

   Answer: (c) Dextranomer/hyaluronic acid is a dual component material. The dextranomer is cross-linked dextran microspheres 80–250 μm in diameter in a gel of hyaluronic acid. The dextranomer, the main bulking agent, is slowly degraded by hydrolysis. The hyaluronic acid represents the transport medium and slowly dissipates over 12 weeks.

   Volume stability over time results from fibroblast migration and collagen ingrowth into the hyaluronic acid matrix between the dextranomer microspheres. Stenberg et al found that histologic samples taken at the time of open reimplantation after failed injection therapy revealed granulomatous reaction of the giant cell type, inflammatory cell infiltration and implant pseudoencapsulation.[3]

4. A 5-year-old female with spina bifida has a poorly compliant bladder with stable hydronephrosis and bilateral grade III vesicoureteral reflux (VUR). Her bladder management includes intermittent catheterization and anticholinergic therapy. Which of the following is true regarding the endoscopic correction of reflux in this patient:

   (a) It has no role in the management of reflux in patients with neuropathic bladders
   (b) Its efficacy is equal to that of patients with nonneuropathic bladders
   (c) Postinjection obstruction is more common than with nonneuropathic bladders
   (d) Bladder management should continue after injection therapy

Answer: (d) Injection therapy in those patients with neuropathic bladders has been shown to be effective. Perez-Brayfield et al describe a success rate of 78%. Neuropathic bladder and injection therapy present a certain set of challenges. Neuropathic bladders often have severe trabeculation and fibrosis, and placement of the injectable material in the correct position and with adequate mound configuration is often more technically challenging. In addition, due to high voiding pressures, neuropathic bladders are at increased risk for mound shifting. These patients should be maintained on a bladder-management regimen including anticholinergic medication and clean intermittent catheterization in order to keep bladder pressures low.[4]

5. A 4-year-old female is found to have recurrent reflux after open ureteral reimplantation. Her parents are interested in the least invasive treatment options. Endoscopic injection in this scenario:

   (a) Is contraindicated
   (b) Has the same efficacy compared to the nonreimplanted ureters

   (c) Requires the same amount of injected material as nonreimplanted ureters
   (d) Should be performed with a full bladder

Answer: (c) Endoscopic correction of reflux after failed reimplantation has been shown to be effective, although less so than for the nonreimplanted ureters. Perez-Brayfield et al describe a cohort of complex patients with reflux after failed open reimplantation, in neurogenic bladders and in duplicated systems. They describe endoscopic correction success rates of 88%, 78% and 74%, respectively. Despite the potential for challenging anatomy, the total volume of dextranomer/hyaluronic acid used and technique performed was similar to patients with uncomplicated reflux. Ectopic ureters with orifices at the bladder neck posed a very challenging problem with success rates of only 14%.[4]

6. A 6-year-old boy undergoes unilateral endoscopic injection therapy for grade III reflux. Excluding treatment failure, the most common complication of endoscopic injection is:

   (a) Development of contralateral reflux
   (b) Postprocedure cystitis
   (c) Ureteral obstruction
   (d) Recurrent hematuria

Answer: (a) The complications of injection therapy include failure, obstruction, and development of contralateral reflux. Elmore et al and Menezes et al both reported a 10% incidence of new contralateral reflux, with females under 5 years of age being at most significant risk.[5,6] The rate of obstruction for all injectable materials is <1%. Puri et al described the incidence of obstruction requiring open reimplantation of PTFE to be 0.33%.[7] Vandersteen et al reported similar results for dextranomer/hyaluronic acid with an obstruction rate of 0.6% per ureter.[8] The development of recurrent hematuria has not been described in any study.

7. Reasons for failure of injection therapy include all of the following except:

(a) Technical difficulty with the injection
(b) Material properties
(c) Presence of urinary tract infection (UTI)
(d) Bladder dynamics

Answer: (c)   Many factors can affect the efficacy of injection therapy. Technical difficulties due to challenging ureteric anatomy by the presence of duplication, bladder trabeculation or diverticula are the most common. Material properties and volume injected also play a role in regard to migration and absorption. Additionally, patients with abnormal bladder dynamics and increased voiding pressures are at increased risk for mound shifting. While the rates of cystitis and febrile UTIs following endoscopic injection are 6% and 0.75%, respectively, there is currently no evidence at this time relating the presence of UTI to treatment failure.[9]

8. A 6-year-old female undergoes cystoscopy and open reimplantation after failed injection therapy for grade IV reflux. The most likely finding of the ureteral orifice at the time of cystoscopy is:

(a) Shifting of mound
(b) Volume loss
(c) Shifting and volume loss
(d) Normal appearance at the ureteral orifice

Answer: (a)   In a study by Diamond et al, of a total of 57 ureters, the most common finding in patients with failed injection of autologous chondrocytes was mound shifting (35%), followed by shifting and volume loss (25%), isolated volume loss (13%), and normal appearing mound (11%). Similar technical failures have been described in collagen, PTFE, and dextranomer/hyaluronic acid.[10]

9. The most common direction for mound shifting is:

(a) Laterally and superiorly
(b) Toward the bladder neck

(c) Cross-trigonal
(d) Proximally into the ureter

Answer: (b)   The most common direction of mound shift is medially and caudally towards the bladder neck. Studies have shown that autologous chondrocytes, PTFE, and dextranomer/hyaluronic acid all shift toward the bladder neck if shifting occurs. Diamond et al describe distally shifted mound in 75% of their technical failures.[10] The mechanism of shifting is thought to be due to the bladder contraction creating pressure gradient toward the bladder neck. Capozza et al found an association between mound shift and those patients with voiding dysfunction symptoms. Twenty-five of 27 patients with treatment failure had voiding dysfunction symptoms including frequency, urgency, and incontinence.[11]

10. Concern for PTFE particle migration after injection therapy is related to particles being less than:

(a) 50 μm
(b) 500 μm
(c) 80 μm
(d) 8 μm

Answer: (c)   PTFE is a chemically inert substance with particle size ranging from 4 to 100 μm; 90% of particles are <40 μm. Concern for migration of PTFE is based upon the fact that macrophages are able to engulf particles <60 μm. Once engulfed, PTFE is unable to be degraded, resulting in cell death. As the macrophage dies the PTFE particles are freed and potentially initiate the formation of a granuloma. Additionally, those particles can theoretically migrate to other organs, including lymph nodes, lung and brain tissue. Therefore, the optimal size of particles is larger than that which can be engulfed by macrophages, so the ideal size is >80 μm.

References

1. Kirsch AJ, Perez-Brayfield M, Smith EA, Scherz HC. The modified STING procedure to correct vesicoureteral reflux: improved results with submucosal implantation with the intramural ureter. J Urol 2004; 171: 2413–16.

2. Leonard MP, Decter A, Hills K, Mix LW. Endoscopic subureteral collagen injection: are immunological concerns justified? J Urol 1998; 160: 1012–16.

3. Stenberg A, Larsson E, Lackgren G. Endoscopic treatment with dextranomer/hyaluronic acid for vesicoureteral reflux: histological findings. J Urol 2003; 169: 1109–13.

4. Perez-Brayfield M, Kirsch AJ, Hensle TW et al. Endoscopic treatment with dextranomer/hyaluronic acid for complex cases of vesicoureteral reflux. J Urol 2004; 172: 1614–16.

5. Elmore JM, Kirsch AJ, Lyles RH et al. New contralateral vesicoureteral reflux following dextranomer/hyaluronic acid implantation: incidence and identification of a high risk group. J Urol 2006; 175: 197–100; discussion 1100–1.

6. Menezes M, Mohanan N, Haroun J et al. New contrateral vesicoureteral reflux after endoscopic correction of unilateral reflux – is routine contralateral injection indicated at initial treatment? J Urol 2007; 178: 1711–13.

7. Puri P, Granata C. Multicenter survey of endoscopic treatment of vesicoureteral reflux using polytetrafluoroethylene. J Urol 1998; 160: 1007–11; discussion 1038.

8. Vandersteen DR, Routh JC, Kirsch AJ et al. Postoperative ureteral obstruction after subureteral injection of dextranomer/hyaluronic acid copolymer. J Urol 2006; 176: 1593–5.

9. Elder JS, Diaz M, Caldamone AA et al. Endoscopic therapy for vesicoureteral reflux: a meta-analysis. I. Reflux resolution and urinary tract infection. J Urol 2006; 175: 716–22.

10. Diamond DA, Caldamone AA, Bauer SB, Retik AB. Mechanisms of failure of endoscopic treatment of vesicoureteral reflux based on endoscopic anatomy. J Urol 2003; 17: 1556–8; discussion 1559.

11. Capozza N, Lais A, Matarazzo E et al. Influence of voiding dysfunction on the outcome of endoscopic treatment for vesicoureteral reflux. J Urol 2002; 168: 1695–8.

Basic science of the urinary bladder

47

Scott R Manson

(Based on chapter written by Armando J Lorenzo and Darius J Bägli)

1. Normal function of the urinary bladder can best be described as:

   (a) An active neuromuscular process
   (b) A passive function to accommodate filling of the bladder
   (c) Dynamically responsive to changing physical and mechanical conditions
   (d) All of the above

   Answer: (d)   The urinary bladder is a unique organ that demonstrates a remarkable integration of neuromuscular, mechanical, and physical properties to perform its function. Bladder contraction is largely an active neuromuscular process. Bladder filling is thought to represent a largely passive phenomenon which can also be modulated by changes in the neuromuscular properties of the bladder in order to maintain low intravesical pressure. Disruption of the molecular mechanisms underlying any of these normal bladder functions places both continence and renal function at risk.

2. Development of the bladder smooth muscle layer from the mesenchyme of the urogenital sinus is dependent upon:

   (a) Cell–cell interactions
   (b) Cell–matrix interactions
   (c) Mechanical stimulation
   (d) All of the above

   Answer: (d)   Normal prenatal bladder development results from a complex interaction of developing cells with the extracellular matrix, other cells, and the presence of appropriate mechanical stimulation which combine to promote the differentiation of developing smooth muscle cells.

3. Contraction of the bladder smooth muscle layer during filling and emptying of the bladder is primarily mediated by _____ upon stimulation by _____ whose concentration gradients are dependent upon _____ levels:

   (a) Actin–myosin; sodium; adenosine triphosphate (ATP)
   (b) Actin–myosin; calcium; ATP
   (c) Microtubules; calcium; ATP
   (d) Microtubules; calcium; guanine triphosphate (GTP)

   Answer: (b)   In regulating the filling and emptying of the bladder, contraction of the bladder smooth muscle cell is mainly the result of contractile forces generated by actin and myosin following phosphorylation of myosin light chain by calcium-dependent kinases. Calcium is maintained in intracellular stores by ATP-dependent calcium pumps; upon neurostimulation, calcium is released from these stores to stimulate the contractile apparatus.

4. Mechanotransduction can best be described as:

   (a) The process by which neurostimulation is transduced into mechanical forces in muscle contraction

(b) The process by which physical forces are converted into biochemical signals and then integrated into a cellular response

(c) A process involved in stimulating hypertrophy and hyperplasia in the bladder in response to an increased mechanical load on the bladder wall

(d) (b) and (c)

(e) All of the above

Answer: (d) The process of converting physical forces into biochemical signals and integrating these signals into a cellular response is known as mechanotransduction. This is an important concept in bladder development and in the response of the bladder to numerous physiologic and pathologic stimuli.

5. Which of the following processes may be involved in the remodeling of the bladder in response to physiologic and pathologic stimuli?

(a) Changes in the degradation of extracellular matrix proteins

(b) Changes in the synthesis of extracellular matrix proteins

(c) Changes in the behavior of bladder smooth muscle cells as a result of the altered composition in extracellular matrix proteins

(d) (a) and (b)

(e) All of the above

Answer: (e) As the bladder develops, or adapts to different stimuli, changes in both matrix production and degradation result in remodeling of the extracellular matrix in the bladder. Since the behavior of bladder smooth muscle cells is closely tied to their physico-mechanical environment, these changes may result in further changes in the behavior of bladder smooth muscle cells (i.e. proliferation, differentiation).

6. The primary neurotransmitter receptors described in activation of contractions of the detrusor muscle are:

(a) The muscarinic receptors

(b) The purinergic receptors

(c) The adrenergic receptors

(d) None of the above

Answer: (a) Innervation of the detrusor muscle is primarily controlled by the muscarinic receptors. However, both purinergic and adrenergic receptors have been described to play a role in innervation of the human bladder, particularly in developmental and pathologic states.

7. As knowledge of the basic science of the bladder increases, we can expect:

(a) The identification of potential pharmacologic targets for the treatment of bladder diseases

(b) An improvement in the early diagnosis of bladder diseases

(c) An improvement in the development of tissue engineering approaches to the treatment of bladder diseases

(d) An increasing awareness for the complexity of the biology of the bladder

(e) All of the above

Answer: (e) Recent times have witnessed a changing view of the bladder from a simple organ to a complex biological system that is responsive to physiologic and pathologic stimuli. Basic science research of the underlying molecular signaling cascades which regulate bladder physiology has already led to a better understanding of the bladder and new potential modes of treatment, and this should continue with further study of the bladder.

Basic science of prostatic development

48

Ellen S Shapiro

1. The endodermal urogenital sinus is derived from the:

   (a) Allantois
   (b) Vitelline duct
   (c) Terminal hindgut
   (d) Cloacal membrane
   (e) Ureteral bud

   Answer: (c)   The prostate develops from the endodermal urogenital sinus (UGS) which is derived from the terminal end of the hindgut or "cloaca", which is Latin for sewer. Septation of the cloaca by the urorectal septum begins at about 28 days of gestation.[1] The rectum and primitive UGS form by the 44th day. The primitive UGS proximal to the mesonephric duct develops into the vesicourethral canal, whereas the region distal of the mesonephric duct becomes the definitive UGS. The UGS adjacent to the bladder (pelvic urethra) differentiates into the lower portion of the prostatic and membranous urethra.[2]

2. Testosterone production by the fetal testis peaks at:

   (a) 8 weeks
   (b) 10 weeks
   (c) 13 weeks
   (d) 16 weeks
   (e) 18 weeks

   Answer: (c)   Prostate growth and development are dependent on androgen production by the fetal testes, which begins at about the 8th week of gestation.[3] Unlike development of the Wolffian duct (WD) derivatives, which are dependent solely on testosterone, the differentiation of the UGS is dependent on the 5α reduced form of testosterone, dihydrotestosterone (DHT). DHT is essential for the growth and development of the prostate.[3-6] By 10 weeks, the prostatic ductal network develops from solid epithelial outgrowths, or prostatic buds, which evaginate from the endodermal UGS immediately below the bladder and penetrate into the surrounding urogenital mesenchyme (UGM).[5] The prostatic ducts rapidly lengthen, arborize and canalize. By 13 weeks, 70 primary ducts are present and exhibit secretory cytodifferentiation.[7]

3. Which of the following is not characteristic of 5α-reductase deficiency syndrome:

   (a) Normal vas deferens
   (b) Persistent Müllerian ducts
   (c) Severe penoscrotal hypospadias
   (d) A vaginal pouch
   (e) Normal testes

   Answer: (b)   The 5α-reductase deficiency syndrome is a form of autosomal recessive male pseudohermaphroditism characterized by severe penoscrotal hypospadias, a blind vaginal pouch, and normal testes with normal epididymes, vasa deferentia, and seminal vesicles.[8] The ejaculatory ducts terminate in the blind-ending vagina, and the prostate is small or undetectable.

4. In the fetal prostate, 5α-reductase expression is never observed in the:

    (a) Urogenital epithelium
    (b) Prostatic buds
    (c) Posterior lobe ductal epithelium
    (d) Ejaculatory duct stroma
    (e) Ventral stroma

    Answer: (c) Shapiro et al have shown androgen receptor expression in the stroma and luminal epithelium of the UGS of the developing human prostate as early as 7 weeks, while 5α-reductase expression is observed only in the prostatic stroma at 7 weeks and in the basal layer of the UGS epithelium at 9 weeks.[9] Regional 5α-reductase expression varies from 7 to 16 weeks, with increasing expression observed in a caudal to cranial direction at every gestational age. Diminished expression occurs after 18–20 weeks. The most posterolateral stroma and the ductal epithelium in the posterior prostatic lobe never express 5α-reductase. The lateral lobes show distal ductal epithelial expression, while the ducts emanating from above the ejaculatory ducts (EDs) express 5α-reductase in their proximal and distal ductal epithelium. These localization studies support the notion that DHT serves largely as a signal amplification for prostatic development and is directly associated with the distance the target tissue is from the testicular androgen source.[9,10]

5. When tissue recombination experiments combine adult bladder epithelium (BLE) with male urogenital mesenchyme, the following structure forms:

    (a) Vagina
    (b) Prostatic ducts
    (c) Seminal vesicle
    (d) Smooth muscle
    (e) Ejaculatory ducts

    Answer: (b) Tissue recombinant experiments have been used to examine epithelial–mesenchymal interactions on the differentiation and organization of prostatic SM.[11] Experiments combined adult prostatic epithelium (PRE) with UGM or seminal vesicle mesenchyme (SVM) or BLE with UGM or SVM. Prostatic ducts developed in all tissue recombinants when UGM was used with either epithelium. SM cells also organized into sheets resembling prostate. When SVM was combined with either epithelium, the prostatic ducts were surrounded by thick SM cells resembling seminal vesicle. The SM was unorganized in grafts of SVM or UGM. These experiments suggest that male UGM dictates spatial organization, but SM differentiation is induced by epithelium. Urothelium may also direct the organization of SM tissue, since urothelium is thought to be a potent inducer of SM differentiation. Cunha[12] has shown that the proximal segments of prostatic ducts near the urethra express urothelial membrane antigen and have associated thick layers of SM cells surrounding them. All of these tissue recombinant experiments show that interactions between the mesenchyme and epithelium are reciprocal.

References

1. Stephens FD. Congenital Malformation of the Urinary Tract. New York: Praeger Publishers, 1993.
2. Hamilton WJ, Mossman HW. The urogenital system. In: Human Embryology: Prenatal Development of Form and Function, 4th ed. New York: Macmillan, 1976; 201.
3. Siiteri PK, Wilson JD. Testosterone formation and metabolism during male sexual differentiation in the human embryo. J Clin Endocrinol Metab 1974; 38: 113.
4. Cunha GR. Epithelio-mesenchymal interactions in primordial gland structures which become responsive to androgenic stimulation. Anat Rec 1972; 172: 179.
5. Imperato-McGinley J, Binienda Z, Arthur A et al. The development of a male pseudohermaphroditic rat using an inhibitor of the enzyme 5α-reductase. Endocrinology 1985; 116: 807.
6. Raghow S, Shapiro E, Steiner MS. Immunohistochemical localization of TGF-alpha and TGF-beta during early human fetal prostate development. J Urol 1999; 162: 509–513.

7. Lowsley OS. The development of the human prostate gland with reference to the development of other structures at the neck of the urinary bladder. Am J Anat 1912; 13: 299–346.

8. Imperato-McGinley J, Guerrero L, Gautieer T et al. Steroid 5α-reductase deficiency in man. An inherited form of pseudohermaphroditism. Science 1974; 186: 1213.

9. Shapiro E, Tang R, Wang B et al. The expression of 5α-reductase and the androgen receptor in the human fetal prostate. J Urol 1996; 155: 534 (Abstract).

10. Mahendroo MS, Cala KM, Hess DL, Russell DW. Unexpected virilization in male mice lacking steroid 5α-reductase enzymes. Endocrinology 2001; 142: 4652–62.

11. Cunha GR, Battle E, Young P et al. Role of epithelial-mesenchymal interaction in the differentiation and spatial organization of visceral smooth muscle. Epith Cell Biol 1992; 1: 76–83.

12. Cunha GR, Donjacour AA, Cooke PS et al. The endocrinology and developmental biology of the prostate. Endocrine Reviews 1987; 8: 388.

Embryology of the anterior abdominal wall, bladder, and proximal urethra

49

Steven E Lerman, Irene M McAleer, and George W Kaplan

1. The abdominal wall is formed from:

    (a) Concentric closure of the somatopleure
    (b) Entoderm replacing mesoderm
    (c) Mesoderm from the notochord
    (d) Ectoderm
    (e) Three sheets of myeloderm

    Answer: (a) During the first 3 weeks of embryogenesis the anterior abdominal wall is represented by the somatopleure, which forms the ventral surface of the embryonic disk. The somatopleure closes concentrically around the umbilical ring and is invaded by mesoderm, which splits into three muscle layers. (Ch 49, page 733)

2. Problems in embryogenesis of the abdominal wall result in which of the following problems:

    (a) Eagle-Barrett syndrome
    (b) Exstrophy
    (c) Cloacal exstrophy
    (d) (a), (b) and (c)
    (e) None of the above

    Answer: (d) All three problems are considered to arise because of problems with the abdominal wall. The Eagle-Barrett syndrome includes disorganized muscle, presumably because of faulty mesenchyme. Exstrophy and cloacal exstrophy are thought to be produced by rupture of or failure of closure of the lower abdominal wall. (Ch 49, page 734)

3. The cloaca arises from ___ during the ____ week(s) of gestation:

    (a) Endoderm; 5th–7th
    (b) Endoderm; first 3
    (c) Mesoderm; first 3
    (d) Mesoderm; 5th–7th
    (e) None of the above

    Answer: (b) The cloaca arises as a caudal expansion of the endodermal hindgut during the first 3 weeks. (Ch 49, page 735)

4. Separation of the cloaca into separate urinary and fecal tracts results in:

    (a) The trigone
    (b) Ejaculatory ducts
    (c) Cowper's glands
    (d) Rathke's folds
    (e) The perineum

    Answer: (e) Rathke's folds are involved in the separation of the urogenital and fecal tracts. The trigone arises from the urogenital sinus as do the ejaculatory ducts. Cowper's glands arise in the bulbous urethra. The perineum forms after the cloacal membrane ruptures and the urogenital and fecal tracts are separated. (Ch 49, page 736)

5. The bladder develops from:

   (a) Ectoderm
   (b) Mesoderm
   (c) Endoderm
   (d) (a) and (e)
   (e) (b) and (c)

   Answer: (e)   The trigone is initially meso-derm but subsequently fills in with epithelium from the urogenital sinus and is eventually endoderm. The bladder itself forms from endoderm from the urogenital sinus and the detrusor is formed from mesoderm. (Ch 49, page 735)

6. The bladder develops from:

   (a) The urogenital sinus
   (b) Mesoderm of the anterior abdominal wall
   (c) Endoderm
   (d) Ureteral buds
   (e) All of the above

   Answer: (e)   The endoderm forms the primi-tive cloaca which splits to form the urogenital sinus and the rectum. The ureteral buds arise from the mesonephric ducts near their entrance into the urogenital sinus and are then incorporated into the sinus in the trigone. The mesoderm of the anterior abdominal wall is thought to form part of the anterior aspect of the bladder. (Ch 49, page 735)

7. Place the following events in correct chrono-logical order:

   (a) Pronephros involutes
   (b) Urorectal septum descends
   (c) Proximal urethra forms
   (d) Müllerian ducts form
   (e) Wolffian ducts form

      (i)   (a), (b), (c), (d), (e)
      (ii) (a), (b), (e), (c), (d)
      (iii) (a), (b), (c), (e), (d)
      (iv) (a), (d), (c), (b), (e)
      (v) (a), (e), (b), (c), (d)

   Answer: (v)   The pronephros involutes as the mesonephric (Wolffian ducts) form. Then the urorectal septum divides the cloaca into the urogenital sinus and rectum. The proximal urethra forms from the urogenital sinus. The Müllerian ducts form from the Wolffian ducts if there is no testis to produce Müllerian inhibiting factor. (Ch 13, page 231)

Radiologic assessment of bladder disorders

50

Douglas E Coplen

1. The best anatomic and functional assessment of the bladder is obtained with a:

   (a) Voiding cystourethrography (VCUG)
   (b) Nuclear cystogram
   (c) Urodynamics
   (d) Ultrasound
   (e) Computerized tomography (CT)

   Answer: (a)   Fluoroscopic imaging gives the best anatomic detail of the bladder, urethra and ureters (in cases of reflux). While not as accurate as urodynamics with regards to bladder function, the VCUG does give functional information with regards to bladder emptying and the appearance of the bladder outlet during voiding.

2. In pediatric patients the best initial bladder imaging modality is:

   (a) VCUG
   (b) CT
   (c) Magnetic resonance imaging (MRI)
   (d) Ultrasound (US)
   (e) Bladder scan

   Answer: (d)   US is ideally suited for the evaluation of bladder symptoms in children because it is painless and noninvasive. The US can direct other imaging.

3. During a VCUG the best visualization of a ureterocele occurs:

   (a) In early filling
   (b) In mid filling

   (c) In late filling
   (d) During voiding

   Answer: (a)   A ureterocele appears as a filling defect at the bladder base. This is best seen during early bladder filling since it can collapse and actually efface at capacity giving the appearance of a diverticulum. A filling defect in the urethra is occasionally, but not reproducibly, seen during voiding.

4. Superior bladder and pelvic spatial imaging resolution is obtained with:

   (a) US
   (b) CT
   (c) MRI
   (d) VCUG

   Answer: (c)   MRI has the advantage of superior soft tissue resolution when compared to CT and US. Different spin-echo sequences allow delineation of fluid-filled structures from the bladder wall.

5. On bladder US, a dilated distal ureter may be confused with all of the following except:

   (a) Ovarian cyst
   (b) Urachal diverticulum
   (c) Bladder diverticulum
   (d) Uterine duplication with hydrocolpos
   (e) Ureterocele

   Answer: (e)   Cystic structures are frequently identified posterior and lateral to the bladder. Real-time US imaging can usually make a definitive diagnosis. A urachal diverticulum is present at the dome of the bladder and is not in the differential diagnosis.

6. Bladder volume as determined by US is best estimated by the formula:

(a) Length × width × depth

(b) $4/3 \times \pi \times width^3$

(c) $0.7 \times$ length × width × depth

(d) $0.5 \times$ length × width × depth

Answer: (c) The bladder is not a perfect circle or a square. The best formula is $0.7 \times$ length × width × depth.

Urodynamics of the upper and lower urinary tract

Jennifer J Mickelson and William E Kaplan

51

1. A healthy 8-year-old girl was referred to a pediatric urologist with concerns of recurrent urinary tract infections. None of the infections are culture proven. The remaining past medical history is negative and she is not on any medications. Her mother states that she has bowel movements every 2–3 days. Your initial investigation besides a physical exam would include:

   (a) Renal ultrasound
   (b) Magnetic resonance imaging (MRI) of the spine
   (c) Voiding history and voiding diary
   (d) Voiding cystourethrography (VCUG)

   Answer: (c)   An accurate voiding history is most important; the use of a voiding diary may also be helpful. (Page 748)

2. A 12-year-old male developed new onset daytime wetting. He has never been dry at night. Urinalysis and urine glucose are negative. Renal ultrasound is normal and VCUG shows no reflux. Plain film kidney ureter bladder (KUB) showed an abdomen packed with stool and the sacrum could not be well visualized. He has occasional episodes of encopresis, which his parents attributed to constipation. The next investigation which should be ordered is:

   (a) DMSA renogram
   (b) Computerized tomography (CT) abdomen
   (c) Barium enema
   (d) Spinal MRI

   Answer: (d)   Children with both fecal and urinary incontinence should have lumbosacral images. In patients with clearly abnormal studies, spinal MRI is performed. (Page 750)

3. A 14-year-old female presents with multiple culture proven urinary tract infections. Urinalysis in the office is negative. VCUG shows no reflux but a trabeculated bladder. Renal and bladder ultrasound shows no hydro but a thickened bladder wall. A uroflow is performed as the patient complains that it is difficult for her to void. She voids 200 ml, which shows a prolonged, intermittent flow pattern. The best screening parameter from uroflow for bladder function is:

   (a) The shape of the uroflow curve
   (b) The maximum flow
   (c) Average flow
   (d) Total voided volume

   Answer: (a)   In a study of 180 school children age 7–16 years, 98% had a bell-shaped flow pattern. Although the maximum flow, the average flow, and time to maximum flow can be of diagnostic interest, the shape of the flow appears to be the best screening parameter. (Page 752)

4. A 4 kg male newborn is having urodynamic investigation following a diagnosis of an

absent sacrum. He has been voiding well on his own, VCUG is negative for reflux and ultrasound is normal. An 8F urodynamics catheter is used for the study. The urodynamics show a capacity of 29 ml, no unstable contractions but a significantly elevated leak-point pressure. This is most likely due to:

(a) Urethral stricture
(b) A noncompliant bladder
(c) A spinal syrinx
(d) Catheter used for the study is too large

Answer: (d) Male newborns usually require a 5F feeding tube for urodynamic evaluation. We try to take care to avoid overly large catheters in newborns, which can obstruct the urethra and produce an abnormally high leak-point pressures, as fluid tries to leak around the catheter. (Page 753)

5. An 8-year-old girl was referred for problems of infrequent voiding and constipation. Her history is consistent with dysfunctional elimination syndrome. Her imaging studies are normal. A urodynamic investigation was performed which showed bladder capacity of 450 ml and a bilateral grade 1 reflux. Her capacity pressure was 18 cmH$_2$O. Her initial management would include:

(a) Bilateral subureteric Deflux injections
(b) Bladder augment
(c) Bowel management and biofeedback
(d) Bilateral ureteral reimplants

Answer: (c) (Figure 51.12, page 757)

6. A 14-year-old male has a history of spina bifida. He managed his bladder with clean intermittent catheterizations since he was 3 years old. He takes 20 mg of oxybutinin XL in the morning and catheterizes every 2–3 h. At night he uses an overnight drainage bag. Previous urodynamics have shown a low detrussor leak-point pressure and good compliance. Recent spinal MRI is normal. A repeat

study shows his first leak at 68 ml at a detrussor pressure of 41 cmH$_2$O; the leakage was minimal. At capacity his pressure was 60 cmH$_2$O with no reflux. His total capacity was 220 ml. The next step in his management should include:

(a) Bladder augment
(b) Bilateral ureteral reimplants
(c) Addition of an alpha-blocker
(d) Bladder neck reconstruction

Answer: (a) It has been shown in several centers that in the myelodysplastic population, children with leak-point pressures of >40 cmH$_2$O are at greater risk for upper tract damage (hydronephrosis and reflux) than patients who have leak-point pressures <40 cmH$_2$O. (Page 759)

7. Rate of filling in urodynamic testing is determined by the bladder capacity. A medium fill rate is based on which percentage of bladder capacity:

(a) 2%
(b) 10%
(c) 15%
(d) 20%

Answer: (d) Joseph[1] noted that a change in detrussor pressure, as well as maximum detrussor pressure, was adversely affected by increasing the rate of filling from slow (approximately 2% of estimated bladder capacity, 0–10 ml/min) to medium fill (approximately 20% of estimated bladder capacity, 10–100 ml/min). In general, it is recommended to fill at <10 ml/min in children. (Page 754)

8. Examination of pressures in the upper urinary tract can be performed using the Whittaker test. A normal unobstructed ureteral pressure is:

(a) <5 cmH$_2$O
(b) <10 cmH$_2$O

(c) <15 cmH$_2$O

(d) <20 cmH$_2$O

Answer: (c) (Table 51.3 Summary of the Whittaker Test, Page 762)

9. A 10-year-old male is referred regarding a painful perineum. If a postvoid bladder scan was performed prior to the evaluation, you would expected the patient's postvoid residual volume to be:

(a) Negligible

(b) 20% of bladder capacity

(c) 25% of bladder capacity

(d) 35% of bladder capacity

Answer: (d) Estimation of residual urine can be an important clue to overall bladder function. Except in infants, the child's bladder should empty to completion with each void. (Page 752)

10. A 5-year-old male is having urodynamic assessment for symptoms associated with a suspected tethered spinal cord. The cystometrogram (CMG) showed elevated detrusor pressures and multiple unstable bladder contractions at low volumes. The rectal catheter was calibrated appropriately with electromyography (EMG) leads in place. A 6F catheter was used along with a fill rate of 15 ml/min of normal saline. The abnormalities in the exam may be due to:

(a) Filling the bladder too slowly

(b) The use of normal saline as opposed to carbon dioxide gas

(c) Vesicoureteral reflux

(d) Filling the bladder too quickly

Answer: (d) It is not recommended to use carbon dioxide gas for filling. Joseph[1] noted that a change in detrusor pressure, as well as maximum detrusor pressure, was adversely affected by increasing the rate of filling from slow (approximately 2% of estimated bladder capacity, 0–10 ml/min) to medium fill (approximately 20% of estimated bladder capacity, 10–100 ml/min). In general, it is recommended to fill at <10 ml/min in children. (Page 754)

Reference

1. Joseph DB. The effect of medium-fill and slow-fill saline cystometry on detrusor pressure in infants and children with myelodysplasia. J Urol 1992; 147: 444–6.

Neurologic control of storage and voiding

52

Julian Wan and John M Park

1. Norepinephrine is used as a neurotransmitter in which of the following?

    (a) Sympathetic postganglionic synapses
    (b) Sympathetic preganglionic synapses
    (c) Parasympathetic preganglionic synapses
    (d) Parasympathetic postganglionic synapses
    (e) Purinergic synapses

    Answer: (a) Norepinephrine is used in sympathetic postganglionic synapses. Purinergic synapses use peptides such as adenosine triphosphate (ATP) and gamma-aminobutyric acid (GABA). All parasympathetic and sympathetic preganglionic synapses use acetylcholine.

2. Which of the following is *not* correct?

    (a) Alpha-adrenergic receptors in the bladder are concentrated more in the trigone and bladder neck
    (b) Beta-adrenergic receptors in the bladder are concentrated more in the fundus
    (c) Cholinergic receptors of the bladder smooth muscle are primarily nicotinic
    (d) Nitrous oxide is an inhibitory neurotransmitter of urethral smooth muscle
    (e) Neuropeptides modulate signals from afferent sensory nerves

    Answer: (c) Cholinergic receptors of the bladder smooth muscle are primarily muscarinic. There are now five distinct subtypes recognized and this fact is exploited to make more precise acting drugs. Alpha-adrenergic receptors are more concentrated in the bladder neck and base; whereas beta-adrenergic receptors are more concentrated in the fundus. Nitrous oxide is a major inhibitory neurotransmitter. Neuropeptides such as substance P modulate the sensation brought by afferent nerves.

3. Which of the following is correct?

    (a) Pelvic nerves are sympathetic and originate from the caudal end of the lumbar spinal cord
    (b) The parasympathetic postganglionic neurons of the bladder are located next to the lumbar cord
    (c) Hypogastric nerves have somatic, parasympathetic, and sensory fibers
    (d) The pudendal nerve nucleus is in the lateral ventral horn of the sacral spinal cord
    (e) Afferent pathways are unaffected by inflammatory conditions and neuropathy

    Answer: (d) The pudendal nerve nucleus is Onuf's nucleus and it resides in the lateral ventral horn of the sacral spinal cord. Pelvic nerves are parasympathetic and originate from the sacral cord. Parasympathetic postganglionic neurons of the bladder are located within the detrusor wall and in the pelvic plexus. Hypogastric nerves carry sympathetic and sensory fibers. Afferent pathways can change after injury or disease. Unmyelinated c-fibers become more active with inflammation and neuropathy.

4. During urine storage, which of the following statements is most accurate?

   (a) Distention of the bladder decreases afferent nerve activity
   (b) During bladder filling the activity of the rhabdosphincter increases
   (c) During bladder filling, the electromyography (EMG) of the urinary sphincter shows less activity as it is relaxing to help hold more urine
   (d) Squirming and crossing of legs helps a child hold urine by mechanically obstructing the urethra and bladder neck
   (e) Storage occurs without any input from the brainstem or cerebrum

   Answer: (b) The rhabdosphincter increases activity during normal bladder filling as part of the guarding reflex. Distention of the bladder increases afferent nerve activity. It also increases EMG activity of the urinary sphincter. Avoidance maneuvers such as squirming and crossing of the legs are believed to trigger somatic afferent pathways to the pudendal nerve which help inhibit bladder contractions. During storage there are active links between the brainstem and cerebrum and efferent and afferent nerves from the sacral spinal cord.

5. During voiding which of the following is *not* true about micturition?

   (a) During micturition sympathetic and somatic pathways are inhibited
   (b) Parasympathetic pathways inhibit the bladder neck and stimulate the bladder smooth muscle
   (c) Transection of the brain above the brainstem will abolish reflex inhibition of the rhabdosphincter with micturition
   (d) Transection of the spinal cord beneath the brainstem will lead to dyssynergia
   (e) The guarding reflex is inhibited by the pontine micturition center prior to voiding

   Answer: (e) The pontine micturition center signals inhibit the guarding reflex at the start of micturition. Sympathetic and somatic pathways are inhibited during micturition, and allow rhabdosphincter relaxation and bladder contractions. Parasympathetic pathways relax the bladder neck by inhibiting contraction and cause micturition by stimulating bladder smooth muscle contraction. Transection of the brain above the brainstem will not abolish inhibition of the rhabdosphincter during micturition. Transection of the spinal cord below the brainstem disrupts the coordinating influences of the pontine micturition center and will lead to dyssynergia.

6. Voluntary control of voiding depends on all of the following *except*?

   (a) Frontal cortex
   (b) Preoptic region of the hypothalamus
   (c) Brainstem
   (d) Cerebellum
   (e) Paracentral lobule

   Answer: (d) All of the other parts of the brain have been found to have a role in the voluntary control of urine.

7. Which of the following is *true* about maturation of voiding control?

   (a) At birth the neonatal bladder is a complete and effective urine storage vessel
   (b) The primitive voiding reflex of neonates is replaced by the mature micturition reflex by 4 years of age in most children
   (c) Animals such as cats and rats are born innately knowing how to void
   (d) Once maturation changes have occurred, they are permanent and cannot regress
   (e) Downregulation of interneuron to excitatory preganglionic neuron synapses

   Answer: (e) Downregulation of interneuron to excitatory preganglionic neuron synapses, possibly by competition for synaptic space, is thought to be crucial to the maturation process. All of the other choices are incorrect.

8. The chilled water test will demonstrate:

   (a) No effect in normal mature children
   (b) No effect in normal adults
   (c) Bladder contractions in infants under 3 years of age
   (d) Bladder contractions in patients with neuropathic bladders
   (e) (c) and (d)

   Answer: (e)   Cold receptors are mediated by c-fibers. In normal mature children and adults there are inhibitory controls which mask the primitive neonatal reflexes. Infants under 4 years of age will normally have a positive response with involuntary bladder contractions. Likewise, patients with neuropathology will also respond, demonstrating that the loss of an inhibitory control may be an effect of neuropathology.

9. Which of the following are *not* correct?

   (a) As babies develop and mature into toddlers primitive urinary reflexes are supplanted by more mature micturition processes
   (b) The transition in infants is as rapid and abrupt as it is in mammalian animals
   (c) Plasticity of the micturition pathways suggests that reemergence of primitive pathways may explain some forms of neuropathology
   (d) Plasticity of the micturition pathways suggests that voiding dysfunction may be due to incomplete transition to mature pathways or the reemergence of primitive pathways
   (e) There is a period where neither primitive nor mature micturition pathways are clearly preeminent

   Answer: (b)   The transition from more primitive micturition reflexes to more mature pathways is rapid and abrupt in animals such as rats and kittens. In humans this process may take several years and there will be a period of time when neither group of pathways predominate. Voiding dysfunction and neuropathology may be due to the reemergence of primitive pathways or the incomplete transition over to mature micturition processes.

10. Which of the following are correct?

   (a) Nerve endings innervate each individual smooth muscle cell of the human bladder
   (b) Removal or alteration of the innervation results in no lasting changes to bladder histology
   (c) Smooth muscle cells under repetitive stress elaborate greater amounts of myosin and myotropin
   (d) Normal smooth muscle cells propagate excitation by direct neuronal cell-to-cell excitation
   (e) Pathological states may manifest their effects by altering the properties of the extracellular matrix

   Answer: (e)   Nerve endings do *not* innervate each individual smooth muscle cell. Smooth muscles are separated from each other and no direct cell-to-cell excitation has yet been shown. Electromechanical coupling, rather than direct neuronal excitation, propagates detrusor contractions. Repetitive stress to smooth muscle cells results in greater amounts of collagen and elastin being laid down, but not myosin or myotropin. Pathological states often have changes in the relative amounts of the different types of collagen.

Neurogenic voiding dysfunction and nonsurgical management

Richard N Yu and Stuart Bauer

53

1. Which vitamin plays a major role in the prevention of neural tube defects?

   (a) Carotene
   (b) Niacin
   (c) Folic acid
   (d) Riboflavin
   (e) B12

   Answer: (c)   The addition of folic acid supplements to the diet of women of childbearing age has reduced the incidence of spina bifida by >80%. In some cases, despite increased folic acid intake, women may still have a fetus with spina bifida owing to antibodies that develop to folate.

2. Which statement is true about children with a thoracic level myelomeningocele?

   (a) Leg function is usually normal
   (b) Infants with this level lesion often have detrusor–sphincter dyssynergy
   (c) Infants with this level lesion have an underactive detrusor
   (d) Older children tend to have a normal upper urinary tract by ultrasound
   (e) Older children tend to easily achieve urinary continence with just clean intermittent catheterization (CIC) alone

   Answer: (b)   The neurologic lesion produced by a myelomeningocele can be quite variable. The bony vertebral level may not correlate to the exact neurologic level or deficits produced. Children with thoracic level lesions will typically have intact sacral reflex arc function involving the sacral spinal roots. But, they commonly have detrusor–sphincter dyssynergy.

3. Urinary tract deterioration within the first 3 years of life is most likely associated with which of the following factors?

   (a) Detrusor areflexia
   (b) Detrusor–sphincter synergy
   (c) Detrusor–sphinter dyssynergy
   (d) Detrusor overactivity
   (e) Incomplete bladder emptying

   Answer: (c)   Seventy-one percent of newborns with dyssynergic voiding had urinary tract deterioration within the first 3 years of life. Deterioration was noted in only 17% of children with synergic voiding and 23% of children with sphincter denervation. Bladder outlet obstruction is a major contributor to the development of urinary tract deterioration in these children. (Figure 53.2)

4. Credé voiding is best avoided in which of the following conditions?

   (a) The presence of vesicoureteral reflux with a reactive external urethral sphincter
   (b) The presence of vesicoureteral reflux with a severely denervated external urethral sphincter
   (c) The presence of vesicoureteral reflux with a low leak-point pressure

(d) An overactive detrusor with a low leak-point pressure

(e) A compliant bladder with a low leak-point presssure

Answer: (a) Credé voiding should be avoided in children with reflux and a reactive external urethral sphincter. The increased sphincter tone and associated bladder outlet resistance requires higher bladder pressures to expel urine and may aggravate the degree of reflux. Credé voiding can be used in patients with low bladder outlet resistance, which is associated with severe external urethral sphincter denervation, and with a low leak-point pressure on urodynamic studies.

5. When considering an antireflux operation in a child with a myelomeningocele, treating which urodynamic parameter beforehand is thought to be most important for achieving a successful result?

(a) Poor compliance
(b) Presence of detrusor overactivity
(c) A high leak-point pressure
(d) (a) and (b)
(e) (a) and (c)

Answer: (d) Untreated poor bladder compliance and high leak-point pressure may result in persistent reflux after antireflux surgery. Therefore, children who cannot empty their bladder spontaneously should be placed on intermittent catheterization to ensure complete emptying. Anticholinergic medications may be useful in patients with poor detrusor compliance in order to lower storage pressure and improve bladder compliance.

6. All of the following may be an outward physical sign of an occult spinal dysraphism except:

(a) Spinal scoliosis

(b) A subcutaneous mass overlying the thoracic spine
(c) An asymmetric gluteal cleft
(d) A draining pilonidal dimple
(e) One leg slightly longer than the other

Answer: (b) An occult spinal dysraphism includes lipomeningocele, intradural lipoma, diastematomyelia, tight filum terminale, dermoid cyst/sinus, aberrant nerve roots, anterior sacral meningocele, and cauda equina tumor. Physical examination may demonstrate a cutaneous abnormality overlying the lower spine, such as a small dimple or skin tag, tuft of hair, asymmetric gluteal cleft, vascular malformation, or subcutaneous lipoma. The child may also have leg abnormalities from nerve root injury.

7. The conus medullaris normally resides opposite which vertebral body at birth?

(a) Thoracic 11 level
(b) Thoracic 12 level
(c) Lumbar 1 level
(d) Lumbar 2 level
(e) Lumbar 3 level

Answer: (d) Under normal circumstances, the conus medullaris ends just below the L-2 vertebra at birth and recedes upwards to T-12 by adulthood.

8. The conus medullaris normally resides opposite which vertebral body in a normal adult?

(a) Thoracic 11 level
(b) Thoracic 12 level
(c) Lumbar 1 level
(d) Lumbar 2 level
(e) Lumbar 3 level

Answer: (b) Under normal circumstances, the conus medullaris ends just below the L-2 vertebra at birth and recedes upwards to T-12 by adulthood.

9. Which of the following maternal factors may be responsible for sacral agenesis in a newborn child?

   (a) Exposure to progestational agents early in the pregnancy
   (b) Exposure to progestational agents later in the pregnancy
   (c) Early gestation, insulin-dependent diabetes
   (d) Insulin dependency later in the pregnancy
   (e) Maternal exposure to tetrahydrocannabinol

   Answer: (c) Insulin-dependent mothers have a 1% chance of giving birth to a child with sacral agenesis. This condition has been reproduced in chicks that were exposed to insulin during embryogenesis. Maternal drug exposure has also been reported to cause sacral agenesis. However, progestational agents and tetrahydrocannabinol have not been associated with sacral malformation or agenesis.

10. Which statement is true regarding neurogenic bladder dysfunction in children with imperforate anus?

   (a) The Peña operation leads to pelvic nerve injury resulting in bladder dysfunction
   (b) Neurogenic bladder dysfunction is almost never seen in patients with a supralevator level lesion
   (c) Neurogenic bladder dysfunction is fairly common in patients with an infralevator level lesion
   (d) A spinal cord abnormality in association with imperforate anal lesions can be seen in 30% of these children

   (e) The incidence of neurovesical dysfunction is unrelated to the presence of a sacral bony defect

   Answer: (d) The Peña procedure utilizes a posterior, midline approach which was developed for correction of a high imperforate anus while minimizing the risk of injury to the pelvic floor nerves. However, 37% of patients do have long-term problems with fecal incontinence. Neurogenic bladder is more common in patients with supralevator level lesions and is related to the presence of a sacral bony defect. Thirty to 70 percent of children with imperforate anus have a spinal abnormality.

11. Most children with cerebral palsy have what type of lower urinary tract function on urodynamic testing?

   (a) A normally reflexic bladder with bladder sphincter synergy during voiding
   (b) A hyperactive bladder with denervation in the external urethral sphincter
   (c) A hyperactive bladder with bladder sphincter dyssynergy during voiding
   (d) An underactive bladder with denervation in the external urethral sphincter
   (e) An underactive bladder with a normally innervated external urethral sphincter

   Answer: (a) Most children with cerebral palsy have a normally reflexic bladder with bladder–sphincter synergy during voiding and they can develop total urinary control. Urodynamic findings may demonstrate a partial, upper motor neuron lesion type of dysfunction with exaggerated sacral reflexes, detrusor overactivity, and/or detrusor–sphincter dyssynergia.

Diurnal and nocturnal enuresis

54

Rosalia Misseri

(Based on chapter written by Mark Horowitz and Rosalia Misseri)

1. When desmopressin acetate is administered, fluid intake should be adjusted downward in order to:

   (a) Decrease the potential occurrence of water intoxication and hyponatremia
   (b) Decrease overnight urine production
   (c) Decrease urine osmolality
   (d) Avoid hypertension related to its weak pressor activity
   (e) Avoid headache and nausea

   Answer: (a) Desmopressin is an analogue of vasopressin with increased antidiuretic activity without vasopressor activity. The risk of water intoxication and hyponatremia should be discussed with parents prior to starting therapy.

2. A 4-year-old girl who was potty trained at 2 years 7 months is referred for evaluation of primary nocturnal enuresis. Her siblings, 7 and 9 years of age, wet the bed until age 6. She has no daytime urinary urgency, frequency or incontinence. Initial therapy includes:

   (a) Oral desmopressin
   (b) Parental reassurance
   (c) Encourage regular daytime voiding schedules and biofeedback
   (d) Encourage regular daytime voiding schedules and encourage emptying the bladder before bed
   (e) Evaluation for obstructive sleep apnea

   Answer: (d) Approximately 25% of 4-year-old children frequently wet the bed. Though parents should be reassured that the majority of children will outgrow this, simple encour-agement of regular daytime voiding and void-ing before bed may ameliorate the situation.

3. Pathophysiologic mechanisms causing noctur-nal enuresis:

   (a) Are related to abnormalities in the circadian rhythm of antidiuretic hormone secretion
   (b) Are related to nocturnal polyuria
   (c) May be related to poor arousability
   (d) (a) and (c)
   (e) All of the above

   Answer: (e) Nocturnal enuresis may be due to one or all of the above.

4. A healthy child with a normal physical exami-nation and severe nocturnal enuresis refrac-tory to therapy with desmopressin acetate and alarm therapy should be:

   (a) Referred for evaluation by a behavioral therapist
   (b) Evaluated for functional and anatomic bladder abnormalities
   (c) Reassured that approximately 15% will become dry yearly
   (d) Evaluated with a lumbosacral magnetic resonance imaging (MRI) scan
   (e) Referred for evaluation of obstructive sleep apnea

   Answer: (b) Children without a history of behavioral disturbances, cutaneous abnor-malities overlying the lumbosacral spine, and snoring would not benefit from choices (a), (d) and (e). Although it is true that approximately

15% of children with nocturnal enuresis will become dry yearly, consideration of underlying bladder dysfunction, such as small functional bladder capacity and detrusor instability, should be explored as the cause of severe refractory enuresis.

5. Nocturnal enuresis may be treated with all of the following except:

(a) Desmopressin acetate
(b) Alarm therapy
(c) Behavioral modification
(d) Prophylactic antibiotics
(e) Acupuncture

Answer: (d) Desmopressin acetate, alarm therapy, and behavioral modification are the most commonly used therapies for nocturnal enuresis. Alternative therapies such as traditional Chinese acupuncture and laser acupuncture have been used. There is no role for antibiotic prophylaxis in children with primary nocturnal enuresis.

Operations for the weak bladder outlet

55

CD Anthony Herndon
(Based on chapter written by Anthony J Casale)

1. Possible side-effects from medications used to treat an incompetent bladder neck include the following *except*:

   (a) Rhinorrhea
   (b) Palpitations
   (c) Hypertension
   (d) Headaches
   (e) Anxiety

   Answer: (a)   Alpha-agonist medication is the primary medical treatment of the incompetent bladder neck; complications include palpitations, headache, anxiety and hypertension.

2. Which population is least likely to experience success with a urethral/bladder neck sling procedure:

   (a) Nonambulatory male
   (b) Combined with a bladder augmentation
   (c) Ambulatory male
   (d) Ambulatory female
   (e) Combined with another bladder neck procedure such as a Young-Dees and augmentation

   Answer: (c)   Of the above options, the ambulatory male patient historically is the most difficult patient to achieve continence after a urethral sling procedure.

3. Potential complications following placement of the artificial urinary sphincter (AUS) include:

   (a) Vaginal obstruction
   (b) Urethral erosion
   (c) Difficulty with catheterization
   (d) AUS infection
   (e) Detrusor decompensation with the need for augmentation

   Answer: (a–e)   All of the above listed complications may result after placement of the AUS. Approximately one-third of patients will require bladder augmentation after placement of the AUS.

4. Of the following bladder neck procedures, which one is most likely to allow volitional voiding:

   (a) Young-Dees-Leadbetter
   (b) Kropp
   (c) Pippi Salle
   (d) AUS
   (e) Urethral/bladder neck sling

   Answer: (d)   Out of the above listed options, volitional voiding is most expected in patients after placement of the AUS. In fact, the ideal patient appears to be one in whom the bladder dynamics are normal (i.e. female epispadias).

Bladder augmentation: current and future techniques

56

Jennifer J Mickelson, Bradley P Kropp, and
Earl Y Cheng

---

1. Gastrocystoplasty is an appropriate form of augmentation for patients in renal failure because:

   (a) Hyperchloremic hypokalemic metabolic acidosis occurs
   (b) It reduces metabolic acidosis by inducing a metabolic alkalosis
   (c) It absorbs more chloride
   (d) It improves renal function

   Answer: (b)   Gastrocystoplasty is a better option for renal failure patients because it induces a hypochloremic hypokalemic metabolic alkalosis. This results in less electrolyte disturbance for this vulnerable patient group. (Table 56.1, page 872)

2. Antireflux surgery should be considered in patients undergoing augmentation if:

   (a) Reflux occurs at low intravesical pressure
   (b) There is a history of infection
   (c) The bladder has poor compliance
   (d) The patient is prone to constipation

   Answer: (a)   Although reflux has been reported to resolve spontaneously after enterocystoplasty, antireflux surgery should be considered at the time of reconstruction, especially if reflux occurs at low intravesical pressures. (Page 873)

3. The mechanism of the metabolic acidosis seen in bladder augmentation with ileum is due to:

   (a) Increased chloride secretion
   (b) Net bicarbonate reabsorption

   (c) Na^+/K^+ ATPase enzyme activity
   (d) Ammonium (NH_4^+) reabsorption

   Answer: (d)   Metabolic acidosis may develop whenever urine is in contact with ileal or colonic mucosa. The mechanism by which this hyperchloremic metabolic acidosis occurs is related to ammonium (NH_4^+) reabsorption. (Page 876)

4. Regardless of the type of bowel segment, certain reconstruction techniques should always be employed when performing enterocystoplasty. These include:

   (a) Ureteral reimplantation
   (b) Bladder neck reconstruction
   (c) Detubularization and bowel reconfiguration
   (d) Appendicovesicostomy

   Answer: (c)   The goal of bladder augmentation is to provide a large-capacity, low-pressure, urinary reservoir. Detubularization of bowel segments prevents synchronous contractions of circular muscles of the gut. The radius of the reservoir is directly related to the volume. The greater the radius in the augmented bladder the larger pressure low-pressure reservoir this translates to. (Page 879)

5. A 12-year-old female patient with spina bifida is about to undergo bladder augmentation for a noncompliant, small capacity bladder. In addition, she is incontinent of stool. She has between five and six loose bowel

movements per day. Which anatomic bowel segment is most important to preserve for this patient?

(a) Transverse colon
(b) Ileocecal valve
(c) Ileum
(d) Sigmoid colon

Answer: (b) The incidence of bowel dysfunction following enterocystoplasty in all patients is 10–54%. The incidence in the spina bifida population is 20%. Since the overall incidence of bowel problems in children with spina bifida is further increased when the ileocecal valve is removed, this segment should be preserved. (Page 884)

6. A 16-year-old girl has had an augmentation cystoplasty and appendicovesicostomy performed for management of her neurogenic bladder. She catheterizes regularly without difficulty but has persistent problems with recurrent stones. The most common stone composition following enterocystoplasty is:

(a) Calcium oxide monohydrate
(b) Uric acid
(c) Magnesium ammonium phosphate (struvite)
(d) Calcium phosphate

Answer: (c) The risk of stone formation after enterocystoplasty ranges from 7 to 52%. The usual stone composition reported is magnesium ammonium phosphate (struvite), although several others have been reported. (Page 885)

7. A 21-year-old male had an enterocystoplasty created 14 years prior. On follow-up ultrasound there is no hydronephrosis. Video urodynamics show a large-capacity, low-pressure reservoir. He infrequently leaks urine. He catheterizes per urethra. The next most important step in his management is:

(a) Bladder neck procedure

(b) Malone Antegrade Continence Enema (MACE) procedure
(c) Cystoscopy
(d) Appendicovesicostomy

Answer: (c) Although the incidence of tumor formation following enterocystoplasty is unknown, lifelong follow-up with yearly cystoscopy and urine cytologies should be considered beginning 6–10 years after augmentation. (Page 886)

8. An 8-year-old girl with a history of bladder augmentation 2 years ago presents with abdominal pain, distended abdomen, and fever. She last catheterized 2 h ago and obtained, 50 ml of urine. A catheter is placed and 10 ml of cloudy urine is obtained. She has a history of chronic constipation. Routine lab work has been drawn. The next best step in her management is:

(a) Ultrasound
(b) Enemas
(c) Urinalysis and culture
(d) Computerized tomography (CT) cystogram

Answer: (d) It may be difficult to distinguish pyelonephritis from spontaneous bladder perforation. Thus, a standard CT cystogram is recommended in any patient with an augmented bladder who presents with the above symptoms. Although the diagnostic role of a cystogram has been questioned in the past, it is the most specific diagnostic radiographic test. (Page 887)

9. A 16-year-old boy has a gastrocystoplasty. Routine follow-up urodynamics show low amplitude phasic contractions <30 cmH$_2$O. Occasionally he will have episodes of coffee-colored urine that doesn't resolve with increased fluid intake. The next best step in management is:

(a) Bicarbonate supplementation

(b) An angiotensin-converting enzyme (ACE) inhibitor

(c) Anticholinergic medication

(d) H2 receptor blockers

Answer: (d) Hematuria-dysuria syndrome (HDS) is unique to gastrocystoplasty and occurs in one-third of patients. Despite the relatively high incidence of HDS following gastrocystoplasty, most patients respond well either to H2 receptor blockers or proton pump blockers such as omeprazole. (Page 891)

10. Preoperative studies which reliably predict success for autoaugmentation include:

(a) Increased compliance with near-normal bladder capacity

(b) Reduced compliance and increased capacity

(c) Normal compliance and decreased capacity

(d) None – preoperative urodynamic studies do not reliably predict success

Answer: (d) Although it appears that patients with increased compliance and large capacity bladder do better with autoaugmentation, mixed results have been obtained clinically with regards to postoperative symptomatic and urodynamic improvement in the autoaugmented bladder. Evaluation of the available data indicates that there is no direct correlation between preoperative urodynamic findings and success. (Page 892)

Urinary diversion

57

Richard Rink and Mark P Cain

1. The most common complication of a temporary vesicostomy is:

   (a) Urinary tract infection
   (b) Parastomal hernia
   (c) Stomal prolapse
   (d) Dermatitis

   Answer: (c) The most common complications of temporary cutaneous vesicostomy in order of occurrence are: stomal prolapse (9–17%); stomal stenosis (3–12%); peristomal dermatitis (3–14%); stone formation (3–7%); and peristomal hernia (3–4%).

2. A 7-year-old male has a transverse colon conduit created for urinary diversion following radiation and excision of a pelvic rhabdomyosarcoma. He does well until postoperative day 7, when the left ureteral stent is inadvertently removed and he has marked increased drainage from the penrose drain. The creatinine on the fluid is >20 mg/dl. Renal ultrasound shows no hydronephrosis. The best management would be:

   (a) Observation
   (b) Placement of a closed-system percutaneous drain
   (c) Immediate reoperation and left to right transureteroureterostomy
   (d) Percutaneous nephrostomy and antegrade stent placement

   Answer: (d) The most likely explanation is an anastomotic leak, which should be amenable to percutaneous drainage and antegrade stent placement. Placement of a foley catheter in the conduit may also be beneficial to minimize extravasation.

3. The benefits of a loop ureterostomy compared to a Sober ureterostomy include:

   (a) Enables continuous cycling of bladder
   (b) Simpler to close
   (c) More complex to create but lower stenosis rate
   (d) Less prone to upper tract infection

   Answer: (b) The Sober Y-ureterostomy is the only high diversion which guarantees some degree of bladder cycling, but it is much more difficult technically to construct.

4. The indications for a surgically placed open cystostomy tube include all but:

   (a) Extensive lower urinary tract reconstruction
   (b) Urethral or bladder trauma
   (c) Complex hypospadias repairs
   (d) Prior extensive pelvic surgery with bowel and adhesions to dome of bladder

   Answer: (c) All are true except (c). While complex hypospadias repairs may be an indication for cystostomy tube, particularly in the older child, it would nearly always be placed percutaneously rather than as an open procedure.

5. Contraindications for percutaneous nephrostomy tube placement are:

   (a) Thrombocytopenia
   (b) Pyonephrosis
   (c) Fungal bezoar
   (d) Impacted ureteropelvic junction stone

   Answer: (a) Relative contraindications for percutaneous nephrostomy tube placement include thrombocytopenia, solitary kidney, and abnormal renal position which would make placement of the tube dangerous. All the other listed problems are indications for percutaneous tube placement.

6. Intestinal conduit diversion is still occasionally performed in children. All of the following bowel segments except one would be acceptable for conduit creation:

   (a) Jejunum
   (b) Ileum
   (c) Cecum
   (d) Transverse colon
   (e) Sigmoid colon

   Answer: (a) Incontinent urinary diversion is rarely used in children and this type of diversion is generally only considered in those patients that are physically or mentally unable to manage continent diversion. Ileum and colon are the most commonly used bowel segments. Jejunum is unacceptable due to the severe electrolyte disorders which may occur.

7. With respect to incontinent ileal or colon conduit diversion, which of the following complications occur most commonly?

   (a) Urinary leak
   (b) Renal deterioration
   (c) Ureteroenteric stricture
   (d) Renal calculi
   (e) Stomal stenosis/stomal prolapse

   Answer: (e) The complications of ileal or colon conduit diversion include urine leak (3–5%), renal deterioration (15–18%), ureteroenteric stricture (8–9%), renal calculi (5–7%), and stomal problems in >20%.

8. Achieving a nonrefluxing submucosal tunneled ureterointestinal anastomosis is most difficult with which intestinal segment?

   (a) Stomach

   (b) Ileum
   (c) Cecum
   (d) Transverse colon
   (e) Sigmoid colon

   Answer: (b) Because of the thicker muscularis of the stomach wall and the colon, the submucosal ureteral tunneling techniques are more successful than with ileum. With ileal segments, the split-cuff nipple technique or the LeDuc technique have been successful in preventing reflux.

9. As a general rule, the lowest sustained intravesical pressure, either in native bladder or continent diversion, which will lead to a high percentage of patients having upper urinary tract deterioration is:

   (a) 10
   (b) 20
   (c) 30
   (d) 40
   (e) 50

   Answer: (d) Since McGuire's early work it is now well accepted that intravesical pressures must be maintained $<40\,cmH_2O$. Newer studies have suggested that pressures $<40\,cmH_2O$ may be deleterious to the ureter and kidneys, but the current standard is $40\,cmH_2O$.

10. Reconfiguring the intestinal segment from a cylinder to a more spherical shape will accomplish all the following except:

    (a) Improve capacity
    (b) Improve electrolyte abnormalities
    (c) Increase wall tension
    (d) Decrease contractility
    (e) Does not eliminate all bowel contractions

    Answer: (b) Reconfiguring and detubularizing the bowel will improve capacity and dampen contractility, but will not completely eliminate all contractions. Wall tension will be increased by increasing the radius (LaPlace's

Law T=Pr). It will not improve the risk of electrolyte abnormalities.

11. Vitamin B12 deficiency can be caused by and result in which of the following?

    (a) Removal of the sigmoid colon
    (b) Removal of large segments of right colon
    (c) Results in microcytic anemia
    (d) Neuropathy
    (e) Can occur within days of removing the distal 20 cm of ileum

Answer: (d) Vitamin B12 deficiency usually occurs from removing a large segment of the distal ileum. Deficiency leads to megaloblastic anemia and neuropathy. Vitamin B12 stores can last for several years and deficiency would take many years to become manifest.

12. Resection of a large segment of ileum can result in all but one of the following:

    (a) Diarrhea
    (b) Vitamin B12 deficiency
    (c) Steatorrhea
    (d) Hypochloremic metabolic alkalosis
    (e) Increased risk of cholelithiasis

Answer: (d) When ileum is incorporated into the urinary tract it will frequently result in hyperchloremic metabolic acidosis, which is worse in the face of renal insufficiency. When >100 cm of ileum is used risk of steatorrhea, diarrhea, and cholelithiasis increases.

13. A 10-year-old child is undergoing lower urinary tract reconstruction requiring a catheterizable abdominal wall urinary channel and the appendix has been used in a Malone Antegrade Continence Enema (MACE) procedure. What tissue should be used to create the channel?

    (a) Distal ureter with transureteroureterostomy (TUU)

    (b) Continent vesicostomy
    (c) Reconfigured ileum
    (d) Stomach tube

Answer: (c) While all the listed tubes have been satisfactorily used, reconfigured ileum (Monti-Yang tube) is the most reliable, with a success rate similar to the "gold standard" appendicovesicostomy. The ureteral tube has a high stomal complication rate and continent vesicostomy is the worst, with a stomal stenosis rate of 40%. The reimplanted stomach tube has a high risk of skin excoriation.

14. Which form of continent urinary reservoir is most likely to result in severe hypokalemia?

    (a) Koch pouch
    (b) Indiana pouch
    (c) Ileal augmentation and catheterizable channel
    (d) Ureterosigmoidostomy
    (e) Penn pouch

Answer: (d) Ureterosigmoidostomy may lead to profound hypokalemia. Ileal segments will reabsorb some of the potassium when exposed to high levels in the urine, but colon will not.

15. Which bowel segment when incorporated into the urinary tract is most likely to result in hyperkalemia?

    (a) Stomach
    (b) Jejunum
    (c) Ileum
    (d) Colon

Answer: (b) Stomach, ileum, and colon are all associated with hypokalemia, but jejunum will result in hyponatremic, hypochloremic, hyperkalemic metabolic acidosis.

The Malone Antegrade Continence Enema procedure

58

Martin A Koyle

(Based on chapter written by Martin A Koyle and Padraig SJ Malone)

1. The highest success rate utilizing the Malone Antegrade Continence Enema (MACE) technique is in:

   (a) Spina bifida
   (b) Anorectal abnormalities
   (c) Downs syndrome
   (d) Hirshspung's disease
   (e) Functional constipation

   Answer: (d) In a survey performed by Malone and Curry[1] of British Association of Paediatric Surgeons (BAPS) members, over 300 cases were collated and success was dependent on the original diagnosis.

2. Quality of life in patients in patients who have undergone the MACE procedure is lowest in:

   (a) Cerebral palsy with poor upper extremity coordination
   (b) Imperforate anus after Soave procedure
   (c) Transverse myelitis with residual bowel dysfunction only
   (d) Hirshprung's disease with residual mega-colon
   (e) Wheelchair-bound spina bifida

   Answer: (e) Malone,[2] using a quality of life score where 5 was perfect, found that wheelchair-dependent children with spina bifida had lower scores than ambulatory patients.

3. A left-sided MACE should be strongly considered in patients with:

   (a) Severe constipation
   (b) Short gut syndrome

   (c) A lax pelvic floor
   (d) Bile salt diarrhea
   (e) Megacolon

   Answer: (a) Mouriquand[3] and others have strongly advocated the virtues of distal placement of the MACE procedure in those with severe constipation, with a spastic pelvic floor. Liloku[4] and Churchill[5] reported shorter washout times when a left-sided MACE was performed.

4. When performing MACE irrigation, the irrigant containing which of the below is associated with potential life-threatening complications:

   (a) Free tap water
   (b) Hypotonic saline
   (c) Go Lytely
   (d) Phosphate
   (e) Magnesium

   Answer: (d) Although in North America tap water is primary irrigant utilized and has a safe profile, phosphate enemas are utilized more commonly in Europe and have been associated with potentially fatal toxicity. Thus, if such a regimen is used, failure of one enema to produce a return, should not be followed by a second phosphate enema.[6]

5. The most common complication related to the MACE procedure is:

   (a) Stoma incontinence
   (b) False passage of the channel
   (c) Stoma stenosis

(d) Pain on infusion

(e) Stoma prolapse

Answer: (c)   Both Denver[7] and Southampton[8] series yielded similar results showing that stoma continence was present in about 98% of patients but stenosis occurred in about 20–30% of patients.

6. The ideal patient for consideration on the MACE procedure should be:

    (a) >5 years of age

    (b) Female

    (c) Right-hand dominant

    (d) Wheelchair bound

    (e) Devoid of prior abdominal surgery

Answer: (a)   The ideal patient is >5 years of age, motivated, tried and failed all conservative nonsurgical therapy, and have a diagnosis of neuropathic bowel, anorectal malformation or Hirschprung's disease.[4]

7. In the absence of an intact appendix, the MACE procedure:

    (a) Should only be approached laparoscopically (LACE)

    (b) Is contraindicated

    (c) Is likely to fail

    (d) Should be performed on the left side

    (e) Can be performed utilizing the Monti technique

Answer: (e)   There are many options including Chait tubes/Mic-Key buttons, colonic extension or flaps which can successfully be utilized when the appendix is deficient or absent. Sugarman suggests the Monti technique as the procedure of choice in such scenarios.[10]

8. Success with the establishment of a MACE channel should be:

    (a) Readily assessable before discharge from hospital

(b) Less likely if concurrent urinary tract reconstruction has been undertaken

(c) Predictable and occur within 30 minutes of irrigant instillation

(d) May take as long as 6 months to occur

(e) Best when the appendix is used

Answer: (c)   It may take up to 6 months for a steady state to occur and hence success to be determined in patients who have under gone the MACE procedure, and depends on underlying condition, bowel motility, patient and parental motivation, and ability to deal with "trial and error".

9. Most rapid mean washout times when a MACE procedure has been performed are when it is:

    (a) Placed on the left side

    (b) Placed in the transverse colon

    (c) In situ appendix

    (d) Performed using a button or Chait tube in the cecum

    (e) Performed using minimally invasive laparoscopic techniques

Answer: (a)   The mean washout time for right-sided MACEs in situ, or right sided, is >30 min, whereas this can be reduced significantly, especially in those with constipation, when a left-sided MACE is performed.[12]

10. A 10-year-old boy with history of cured spinal cord neuroblastoma is incontinent of stool and urine. Continent reconstruction of both systems is strongly considered if:

    (a) The appendix is intact and can be split for dual stomas

    (b) A colostomy is considered as a primary option

    (c) He is not wheelchair bound

    (d) He is highly motivated

    (e) Had stage IV S neuroblastoma

Answer: (d)   Although being wheelchair bound may be associated with a less successful outcome, being >5 years of age and highly motivated is the key to successful outcome. The appendix may be split in selected circumstances but is not absolutely necessary for either the MACE or Mitrofanoff technique. Initial tumor stage is irrelevant. In a child being considered for urinary continence reconstruction, it is paramount that the patient is assessed for fecal continence as well, as simultaneous reconstruction does not jeopardize the success of either individual component.

References

1. Curry JL, Osborne A, Malone PS. The MACE procedure: experience in the United Kingdom. J Pediatr Surg 1997; 34: 338–40.
2. Malone PS, Wheeler RA, Williams JE. Continence in patients with spina bifida: long term results. Arch Dis Child 1994; 70: 107–10.
3. Mouriquand P, Mure PY, Feyaerts A et al. The left Monti Malone. BJU Int 2000; 85: 65.
4. Liloku RB, Mure PY, Braga L et al. The left Monti-Malone procedure: preliminary results in seven cases. J Pediatr Surg 2002; 37: 228–31.
5. Churchill BM, De Ugarte DA, Atkinson JB. Left-colon antegrade continence enema (LACE) procedure for fecal incontinence. J Pediatr Surg 2003; 38: 1778–80.
6. Aksnes G, Dieseth TH, Heleseth A et al. Appendicostomy for antegrade enema: effects on somatic and psychosocial functioning in children with myelomeningocele. Pediatrics 2002; 109: 484–9.
7. McAndres HF, Malone PS. Continent catheterizable conduits: which stoma, which conduit and which reservoir? BJU Int 2002; 89: 86–9.
8. Barqawi A, DeValdenebro M, Furness PD 3rd, Koyle MA. Lessons learned from stomal complications in children cutaneous catheterizable continent stomas. BJU Int 2004; 94: 1344–7.
9. Curry JL, Osborne A, Malone PS. How to achieve a successful Malone antegrade continence enema. J Pediatr Surg 1998; 33: 138–41.
10. Sugarman ID, Malone PS, Terry TR, Koyle MA. Transversely tubularized ileal segments for the Mitrofanoff or Malone antegrade continence enema procedures: the Monti principle. BJU 1998; 81: 253–6.
11. Wedderburn A, Lee RS, Denny A et al. Synchronous bladder reconstruction and antegrade continence enema. J Urol 2001; 165: 2392–3.
12. Kajbafzadeh AM, Chubak N. Simultaneous Malone antegrade continent enema and Mitrofanoff principle using the divided appendix: report of a new technique for prevention of stoma complications. J Urol 2001; 165: 2404–9.

Minimally invasive approaches to lower urinary tract reconstruction

59

Christina Kim and Steven G Docimo

1. Which of the following is an anticipated benefit of laparoscopic-assisted bladder reconstruction over open reconstruction:

   (a) Improved bladder capacity
   (b) Lower risk of stone formation
   (c) Lower risk of intra-abdominal adhesions
   (d) Lower risk of stomal stenosis
   (e) Improved continence]

   Answer: (c) Laparoscopic surgery is associated with a significantly lower risk of developing intra-abdominal adhesions in both children and adults. The other outcomes are not dependent on the approach. (Page 958)

2. A contraindication to laparoscopic-assisted bladder augmentation is:

   (a) Prior abdominal surgery
   (b) Poor adherence to a catheterization regimen
   (c) Ventriculoperitoneal shunt
   (d) Nonneurogenic bladder dysfunction
   (e) Need for a Mitrofanoff stoma

   Answer: (b) The majority of laparoscopic-assisted reconstructions have been performed in patients with prior abdominal surgery. Ventriculoperitoneal shunt is not a contraindication to laparoscopy. The indications for bladder reconstruction do not limit the approach, whether open or laparoscopic. No bladder reconstruction should be attempted without assurance that the child and/or family will adhere to an emptying schedule. (Page 958)

3. The most compelling argument against performing laparoscopic bladder autoaugmentation in a child with poor bladder volume and compliance is:

   (a) Low long-term success of autoaugmentation in this scenario
   (b) Converting an extraperitoneal operation to a transperitoneal operation
   (c) High risk for bladder perforation
   (d) Expected difficulty dissecting detrusor off of the bladder mucosa
   (e) High risk of bladder calculi

   Answer: (a) Bladder autoaugmentation is an ideal operation for adaptation to laparoscopy. Unfortunately, the long-term results, especially in children with low bladder volume, have been poor. The operation can be done transperitoneally or preperitoneally, the risk for bladder perforation and stones is probably lower than for gastrointestinal augmentation, and the dissection of bladder muscle off of detrusor, while potentially difficult, is reasonably accomplished laparoscopically. (Page 959)

4. All of the following are important technical points in laparoscopic ileocystoplasty except:

   (a) Ileal detubularization
   (b) Wide bladder opening
   (c) Tension-free anastomosis
   (d) Adequate postoperative drainage
   (e) Intracorporeal bowel anastomosis

   Answer: (e) Laparoscopic ileal augmentation has been done with both extra- and intracorporeal bowel anastomosis, with little effect on outcome. The others are important to any intestinal bladder augmentation, regardless of approach. (Page 962)

5. Umbilical access as most commonly described for a laparoscopic-assisted bladder reconstruction with appendicovesicostomy:

(a) Incorporates a 3 mm trocar
(b) Is obtained through an open approach after creating a posterior umbilical skin flap
(c) Should not be used in order to preserve umbilicus for stoma
(d) Is best obtained directly through posterior umbilicus with Veress needle
(e) Is enlarged in order to perform the open portion of the procedure

Answer: (b) In the typically described laparoscopic-assisted reconstruction, a posterior umbilical flap is created in order to make a concealed umbilical stoma at the end of the case. Open access is then obtained using a radially dilating 10 mm trocar. The open portion of the procedure is performed through a low incision, usually a Pfannensteil.

Genitourinary rhabdomyosarcoma and other bladder tumors

60

Paul A Merguerian and Antoine E Khoury

(Based on chapter written by Paul A Merguerian, Lisa Cartwright, and Antoine E Khoury)

1. Rhabdomyosarcoma (RMS) is associated with the following syndromes except:

   (a) Neurofibromatosis
   (b) Denys-Drash syndrome
   (c) Beckwith-Wiedemann syndrome
   (d) Li-Fraumeni syndrome

   Answer: (b) RMS may be associated with congenital anomalies including the nervous system and the genitourinary (GU) system. Neurofibromatosis is the most common syndrome in which RMS has been described. The incidence is 0.5% (Intergroup Rhabdomyosarcoma Study-IV study). The disease in these patients is very progressive and it is recommended that patients with RMS and neurofibromatosis be treated with intensive contemporary therapy protocols. Costello syndrome is associated with increased risk of solid tumors including RMS. Other congenital syndromes associated with RMS are Gorlin's basal cell nevus syndrome, Rubinstein-Taybi syndrome, trisomy 21, Beckwith-Wiedemann syndrome, fetal alcohol syndrome, and Li-Fraumeni syndrome. Whereas Wilms' tumor is the most common malignancy associated with Beckwith-Wiedemann syndrome, in the first 7 years of life, RMS, adrenocortical carcinoma, and hepatoblastoma may be seen.

2. Translocation involving chromosome 2 and 13 is associated with:

   (a) Wilms' tumor
   (b) Embryonal RMS (ERMS)
   (c) Alveolar RMS (ARMS)
   (d) Neuroblastoma

   Answer: (c) ARMS reveal a translocation involving chromosomes 2 and 13, t(2,13) (q35;q14). There have also been several reports of translocation involving chromosomes 1 and 13, t(1,13)(p36;q14). In a series of mapping experiments, the chromosome 2 locus disrupted by the t(2;13) was found to be PAX3, and translocation breakpoints were localized to the final intron of the PAX3 gene. The chromosome 13 gene was cloned and found to be a novel widely expressed member of the fork head transcription factor family. Based on homology to this family, the chromosome 13 gene was named FKHR for "fork head in rhabdomyosarcoma". The PAX3–FKHR fusion in ARMS is characterized by rearrangement of chromosomes 2 and 13, t(2,13)(q35;q14), in which the PAX3 gene within band 2q35 is fused with the FKHR gene within band 13q14.

3. PAX3–FKHR fusion is associated with:

   (a) Wilms' tumor
   (b) ERMS

(c) ARMS

(d) Neuroblastoma

Answer: (c)   See explanation in answer 2.

4. The cambium layer is found in which condition:

(a) Neuroblastoma

(b) Wilms' tumor

(c) Botryoid embryonal RMS (BRMS)

(d) Nephrogenic adenoma of the bladder

Answer: (c)   The International Classification of Rhabdomyosarcoma (ICR) criterion for diagnosis of BRMS requires demonstration of a cambium (condensed layer of rhabdomyoblasts) tumor layer underlying an intact epithelium in at least one microscopic field. This microscopic criterion supersedes any gross demonstration of a "grape-like" tumor mass. An extensive degree of rhabdomyoblast differentiation can be evident both in the cambium layer and elsewhere in the tumor. The importance of diagnosing this subtype is evident given its superior prognosis with a 95% 5-year survival.

5. Which variants of RMS have superior prognosis?

(a) ERMS

(b) Spindle-cell ERMS

(c) BRMS

(d) (a) and (c)

(e) (b) and (c)

Answer: (e)   Classic ERMS with a polypoid growth pattern was associated with a more favorable prognosis than the diffuse intramural growth pattern. The 10-year survival for the polypoid tumor was 92% versus only 68% for the diffuse intramural growth pattern. BRMS has a superior prognosis with a 95% 65-year survival. The spindle-cell variant also enjoys a superior prognosis with an 88% 5-year survival rate. This variant occurs exclusively in the paratesticular region, although it can rarely occur at other body sites. ARMS carries a poorer prognosis with only a 53% 5-year survival rate.

6. In a child with pelvic RMS, the presence of posttreatment residual rhabdomyoblasts in the tissue specimen:

(a) Occurs more often in ARMS

(b) Is indicative of a worse prognosis

(c) Their numbers increase with time

(d) Their presence is not an indication for further therapy

(e) None of the above

Answer: (d)   The most difficult assessment by pathologists is the prognostic significance of residual rhabdomyoblasts in posttherapeutic RMS tissue specimens. Studies support the concept that posttherapeutic cytodifferentiation occurs more frequently in BRMS or ERMS (Heyn 1997[1], Coffin 1997[2], Smith et al 2002[3]). In BRMS, cytodifferentiation and decreased proliferation activity were associated with favorable outcome. Unchanged or increased posttherapeutic proliferation activity suggested aggressive biologic potential in ERMS or ARMS.

Smith et al[3] reported on the posttreatment cytodifferentiation and clinical outcome from 19 of 31 IRS-IV cases which were adequate for evaluation. None of the 10 cases with extensive cytodifferentiation (2 BRMS, 8 ERMS) failed, while among the 5 cases with moderate cytodifferentiation, only the 2 ARMS patients failed, and all 4 patients (1 ERMS, 3 ARMS) with mild or no cytodifferentiation failed. The authors concluded that posttreatment cytodifferentiation is more common in both ERMS and BRMS than in ARMS, and postulated that this difference is due to different mechanisms to cellular response to therapy. They also noted that sparse persistent tumor cells in ARMS/BRMS did not appear to affect outcome (Smith et al 2002[3]). Myoglobin is specific for terminally differentiated myocytes, and as such is a useful marker for differentiated tissue in organs such as bladder and prostate, which normally do not contain skeletal muscle.

RMS with persistent well-differentiated rhabdomyoblasts without mitotic activity during and after the completion of therapy demonstrated rhabdomyoblast persistence, but decrease in number with time. All six patients were alive with no evidence of disease 37–233 months after the completion of therapy. The authors conclude that, while the biologic nature of these cells is not known, their presence is not an indication for further therapy (Ortega et al., 2000[4]).

7. The following are all important prognostic factors predicting survival of patients with RMS except:

(a) Age at presentation
(b) Primary site
(c) Clinical group
(d) Tumor size
(e) ICR based on tumor histology

Answer: (a) The significant difference in survival between ERMS and ARMS makes it imperative for the pathologist to accurately diagnose variants of RMS so that the biological course of the disease can be predicted and appropriate therapy initiated.

In 1995, a consensus classification of RMS was published (Newton 1995[5]) that was based on a review of a large number of tumors from IRS-II by 16 international pathologists from eight pathology groups. This produced a classification which was both reproducible and could predict outcome by univariate analysis. A multivariate analysis of this new ICR indicated that a survival model which included the ICR along with known prognostic factors of primary site, clinical group, and tumor size was significantly better at predicting survival than a model with only the known prognostic factors.

8. The incidence of immunopositivity for antisera in RMS diagnostic studies is highest for:

(a) Polyclonal desmin
(b) Monoclonal desmin
(c) Myoglobin
(d) MIC-2

Answer: (a) Polyclonal antidesmin (P-DES) antibody is positive in 99% of RMS specimens. Monoclonal antidesmin (M-DES) antibody was negative in many of the same tumors (38%). Antimuscle specific actin (MSA) antibody was positive in 94% of the RMS. Antimyoglobin (MYO) antibody was positive in 78% and was negative mostly in the less differentiated tumors. Antialpha smooth muscle actin (SMA) antibody reacted positively only in a minority (4%) of embryonal RMS (Qualman 1998[6]).

The current approach at the IRSG Pathology Center in cases where the diagnosis of RMS is in question is to screen the case with immunostaining for three antibodies: P-DES, MSA, and MIC-2; the latter helps to rule out the diagnosis of an extraosseous Ewing's sarcoma/primitive neuroectodermal tumor.

9. A 7-year-old male was found to have a large pelvic tumor extending from the bladder causing bilateral hydronephrosis. Biopsy of the tumor confirmed ERMS. There is no evidence of distant metastasis. What is the clinical group of this tumor?

(a) Clinical group IIIB
(b) Clinical group IIC
(c) Clinical group IIIA
(d) Clinical group IIB

Answer: (c)
Clinical group I   Localized tumor completely resected:

(a) Confined to site of origin
(b) Infiltration beyond site of origin

Clinical group II Microresidual or regional spread:

(a) Localized with micropositive margins, grossly resected
(b) Regional disease with complete resection, most distal nodes negative
(c) Regional disease resected with microresidual or most distal resected nodes involved

Clinical group III Gross residual:

(a) Biopsy only
(b) Gross/major primary resection (>50%)

Clinical group IV Distant metastasis at diagnosis (lung, liver, bone marrow (BM), bone, brain, distant muscle and/or cytology cerebrospinal fluid (CSF), pleural fluid, peritoneal fluid).

10. Transitional cell carcinoma of the bladder in children is usually:

(a) Muscle invasive
(b) Low grade tumor
(c) Has high recurrence rate
(d) Multifocal

Answer: (b) Transitional cell carcinoma of the bladder in children is low grade which seldom recurs. Some of these tumors occur secondary to cyclophosphamide therapy.

In >90% the lesions are solitary. Pathologically, 80% are grade I or papilloma, 20% are grade I–II, and only 3% invasive through the lamina propria. The recurrence rate is low (25%). Cystoscopy allows definitive diagnosis, staging, and treatment of these tumors. Its role in surveillance remains ill defined.

References

1. Heyn R, Newton WA, Raney RB et al. Preservation of the bladder in patients with rhabdomyosarcoma. J Clin Oncol 1997; 15: 69–75.
2. Coffin CM, Rulon J, Smith L et al. Pathologic features of rhabdomyosarcoma before and after treatment: A clinicopathologic and immunohistochemical analysis. Mod Pathol 1997; 10: 1175–87.
3. Smith LM, Anderson JR, Coffin CM. Cytodifferentiation and clinical outcome after chemotherapy and radiation therapy for rhabdomyosarcoma (RMS). Med Pediatr Oncol 2002; 38: 398–404.
4. Ortega JA, Rowland J, Monforte H et al. Presence of well-differentiated rhabdomyoblasts at the end of therpy for pelvic rhabdomyosarcoma: implications for the outcome. J Pediatr Hematol Oncol 2000; 22: 106–111.
5. Newton WAJr, Gehan EA, Webber BL et al. Classification of rhabomyosarcomas and related sarcomas. Pathologic aspects and proposal for a new classification – an Intergroup Rhabdomyosarcoma Study. Cancer 1995; 76: 1073–85.
6. Qualman SJ, Coffin CM, Newton WA et al. Intergroup Rhabdomyosarcoma Study: up date for pathologists. Pediatr Dev Pathol 1998; 1: 550–61.

Exstrophy and epispadias 61

Linda A Baker and Richard W Grady

1. Single-stage reconstruction using the complete primary exstrophy repair technique offers several advantages over staged reconstruction except:

   (a) The possibility to correct the penile, bladder, and bladder-neck abnormalities of bladder exstrophy with one operation
   (b) The ability to achieve urinary continence without bladder-neck reconstruction
   (c) Correction of vesicoureteral reflux at the time of surgery
   (d) Lower complication rates than previous attempts at single-stage reconstruction

   Answer: (c) Complete primary closure affords the above mentioned advantages. However, it is typically performed in the neonatal period which precludes the surgical correction of reflux. (Page 1014)

2. Single-stage reconstruction using the complete primary repair of exstrophy (CPRE) technique relies on the following to achieve urinary continence except:

   (a) Reestablishment of normal anatomic relationships
   (b) Bladder-neck reconstruction at the time of primary surgery
   (c) Osteotomy at the time of single-stage reconstruction
   (d) Simultaneous epispadias repair
   (e) None of the above

   Answer: (b) CPRE involves division of the intersymphyseal band which allows the placement of the bladder and reconstructed urethra deep into the pelvis, and reestablishment of normal anatomy. This relationship will allow bladder cycling and continence, which some believe may preclude the need for a formal bladder-neck repair. (Page 1015)

3. The following postoperative factors have been shown to increase the success of reconstruction for bladder exstrophy except:

   (a) Immobilization with external fixators, Buck's traction, a Spica cast, etc.
   (b) Antibiotic therapy
   (c) Prolonged nil per os (NPO) status or high resin diet to avoid excessive bowel movements which may soil the dressing and cast
   (d) Urinary diversion through ureteral stenting and suprapubic urinary drainage
   (e) Adequate nutritional support

   Answer: (c) Factors recognized to increase success of the initial reconstruction are: use of osteotomies; immobilization; use of postoperative antibiotics; urinary diversion; adequate pain control; avoiding abdominal distention; adequate nutrition; and fixation of urinary drainage catheters. (Page 1013)

4. Single-stage reconstruction using the complete primary exstrophy repair (CPRE) technique can be safely performed because:

   (a) The neurovascular bundles of the corporal bodies lie laterally rather than dorsally on the corporal bodies

(b) The cavernosal bodies and urethral wedge are not actually separated from each other with this technique

(c) The blood supply to the corporal bodies and urethral wedge are independent of each other

(d) The blood supply is quickly reestablished once the components are "reassembled"

(e) (a) and (c)

Answer: (e) The corporal bodies and urethral wedge are separated into three distinct parts with their respective independent blood supply. Dissection should be carried out above Buck's fascia to avoid injury to the laterally placed neurovascular bundle (NVB) on the corpora. The wedge should be wide proximally to assure adequate vascuralization during tubularization of the urethra. (Page 1015)

5. The proximal limits of dissection using the complete primary exstrophy repair (CPRE) technique are:

(a) The intersymphyseal band
(b) The muscles of the pelvic floor complex
(c) The rectum
(d) The corpora spongiosa

Answer: (b) The proximal dissection should include division of the intersymphyseal bands, which is achieved with the penile disassembly. The dissection terminates at the level of the pelvic floor musculature. Failure to reach this point will result in tension on the repair. (Page 1015)

6. Factors that mitigate against using a single stage reconstruction technique for cloacal exstrophy include the presence of:

(a) A large omphalocele
(b) A wide pubic diastasis
(c) A concomitant myelomeningocele
(d) All of the above

Answer: (d) The size of the omphalocele, the size of the hindgut and bladder plates, the

extent of the pubic diastasis, and the extent of other comorbidities such as spina bifida should factor into a decision to proceed with CPRE of cloacal exstrophy. (Page 1036)

7. Complications of the complete primary exstrophy repair (CPRE) technique include:

(a) Myogenic bladder failure
(b) Testicular atrophy
(c) Urethrocutaneous fistula
(d) Hip dislocation

Answer: (c) CPRE should provide bladder cycling which prevents myogenic bladder failure. Notable complications in the largest series include hydronephrosis, hypospadias, bladder-neck urethrocutaneous fistula, partial or complete penile loss. (Pages 1009, 1022)

8. Other commonly affected organ systems associated with cloacal exstrophy include:

(a) Liver
(b) Spine
(c) Ears
(d) Upper gastrointestinal tract
(e) (b) and (c)

Answer: (e) Spina bifida and short gut syndrome are two relatively common organ systems affected by cloacal exstrophy. Other systems may be affected as well. (Page 1003)

9. The cloacal membrane separates the coelemic cavity from the amniotic space during the _____ week of embryogenesis

(a) 1st
(b) 12th
(c) 3rd
(d) 24th
(e) 8th

Answer: (c) The cloacal membrane separates the coelemic cavity from the amniotic space and can be first identified at 2–3 weeks gestation. (Page 1006)

10. Left untreated, most patients with exstrophy will experience:

(a) Incontinence
(b) Urinary infections
(c) Difficulty with sexual intercourse
(d) Inflammation of the bladder plate
(e) All of the above

Answer: (e) Closure of bladder exstrophy is not mandatory but chronic exposure of the bladder urothelium will lead to all of the above mentioned complications. (Page 1009)

Unusual conditions of the bladder, including bladder trauma, urachal anomalies, and bladder diverticula

62

Marc Cendron

1. During embryological development of the bladder:

   (a) The urogenital sinus forms at 12 weeks gestation
   (b) The allantois will form the dome of the bladder
   (c) Histological organization of the bladder will be complete by 12 weeks gestation
   (d) Structural and functional organization is complete by 16 weeks gestation

   Answer: (d) With urine production starting at 9–10 weeks gestation, urine flow into the bladder starts. Filling and emptying (cycling) into the bladder has been documented by prenatal ultrasonography. Histologic studies have shown that the organization of the bladder is complete by 16 weeks gestation.

2. Bladder agenesis:

   (a) Can be associated with survival mostly in males
   (b) Is associated with a high rate of ectopic ureter and dysplastic kidney
   (c) Is invariably associated with stillbirth
   (d) Is an isolated congenital anomaly

   Answer: (b) Failure of bladder development causes the ureters to become incorporated into the urethra, vestibule or Gratner's duct in females or prostatic urethra in male. This, in turn will cause distal urethral obstruction early in development of the upper urinary tract. Dilatation of the ureters and dysplasia of the renal parenchyma are the end result.

3. A 3-year-old girl sustained blunt trauma to the lower abdomen. In the emergency department, she presents with gross hematuria after voiding spontaneously once. On physical examination her abdomen is benign and no orthopedic issues are present. The next step in management is:

   (a) Place a Foley catheter for drainage
   (b) Carry out a cystogram to evaluate for a possible bladder leak
   (c) Obtain an ultrasound or computerized tomography (CT) scan of the abdomen
   (d) Admit for observation

   Answer: (c) The patient may have either bladder contusion or bladder rupture. A CT scan or an ultrasound will reveal thickened, irregular bladder wall with no extravasation of fluid. If bladder rupture has occurred, a collection of extravesical fluid will be observed.

4. A 5-year-old boy is involved in a motor vehicle accident and at the time was wearing a seatbelt. He is suspected of having a rupture of his bladder on CT scan. A cystogram is equivocal. He is admitted for observation and over the next 6h is increasingly uncomfortable with increased abdominal girth and displays peritoneal signs. The next step in management is to:

   (a) Place a Foley catheter
   (b) Obtain STAT serum electrolytes
   (c) Consult general surgery
   (d) Repeat the CT scan

   Answer: (b) Urine electrolytes will show decreased levels of bicarbonate indicative of acidosis. Additionally, with an intraperitoneal bladder rupture increased serum creatinine and potassium will be noted. Hyponatremia may also be reported.

5. During imaging of the bladder for a suspected bladder injury, the most important step is:

   (a) Using intravenous (IV) contrast for the CT scan
   (b) Inserting a Foley catheter and injecting contrast material using a syringe
   (c) Obtaining postdrainage images after bladder emptying
   (d) Obtaining delayed films of the abdomen after CT scan

   Answer: (c) Obtaining bladder drainage films to evaluate for possible extravesical extravasation of contrast material. This can also be obtained after CT scan and retrograde bladder filling.

6. Extraperitoneal bladder rupture can be managed by:

   (a) Simple urethral catheter drainage for 7–10 days

   (b) Suprapubic urinary diversion
   (c) Exploration and closure of the bladder
   (d) Exploration to look for bony spicules if a pelvic fracture has been diagnosed

   Answer: (a) Extraperitoneal bladder rupture can be managed nonoperatively with urethral catheter drainage for 7–10 days with follow-up cystogram to rule out persistent extravasation. Surgical exploration is reserved for cases where more severe injuries have been noted such as pelvic fracture with presence of bony spicules in the bladder wall.

7. Congenital bladder diverticula are associated with the following congenital syndromes except:

   (a) Trisomy 23
   (b) Ehlers-Danlos syndrome
   (c) Williams syndrome
   (d) Menkes syndrome

   Answer: (a) Trisomy 23 is not associated with Down's syndrome. All the other syndromes are known to have presence of bladder diverticula.

8. A patient with Menkes, kinky hair syndrome, is noted to have multiple bladder diverticulae and suffers from recurrent urinary tract infection. The most appropriate management would be:

   (a) Placement of an indwelling Foley catheter
   (b) Surgical excision of the bladder diverticula
   (c) Clean intermittent catheterization
   (d) Chronic antibiotic prophylaxis

   Answer: (c) Clean intermittent catheterization, as this will allow for frequent emptying of the bladder and prevention of urinary stasis.

9. Differential diagnosis of bladder outpouching in the pediatric age group includes all of the below except:

   (a) Bladder ears
   (b) Bladder diverticulum
   (c) Everting ureterocele
   (d) Ectopic ureteral insertion
   (e) Urachal cyst

   Answer: (e)   Urachal cyst is distinct from the bladder and is usually identified by either CT scan or ultrasound between the bladder dome and the umbilicus.

10. A 7-year-old child presents to the emergency department with a tender subumbilical mass with erythema of the skin. A CT scan revealed a urachal cyst. The next step in the management would be:

   (a) Admit for antibiotic therapy and observation
   (b) Discharge on oral antibiotics
   (c) Incision and drainage in the operating room under antibiotic coverage with surgical excision at a later stage
   (d) Surgical excision while on antibiotic coverage

   Answer: (c)   Incision drainage with antibiotic coverage followed by surgical excision once the inflammatory process has subsided. Excision of the cyst and closure of the skin may allow for persistence of the infection.

Posterior urethral valves

63

Stephen A Zderic and Douglas A Canning

1. The end-stage bladder following partial outlet obstruction is best associated with:

   (a) A drop in the extracellular matrix fraction within the bladder wall
   (b) A decline in average smooth muscle bundle size
   (c) Bladder wall hypoxia during bladder filling
   (d) A minimal postvoid residual
   (e) A minimal postobstructive diuresis

   Answer: (c)   Much evidence supports the notion of a bladder wall microcirculation which serves to maintain adequate oxygen tension within the bladder wall during normal filling cycles. Lapides[1] first suggested nearly 40 years ago that outlet obstruction resulted in bladder wall hypoxia, and modern molecular and physiology studies demonstrate he was correct. The cyclic drop in perfusion followed by reperfusion leads to free-radical-mediated damage. Partial outlet obstruction leading to the end-stage bladder is clearly associated with significant increases in smooth muscle bundle size, extracellular matrix deposition, postvoid residual urine, and a postobstructive diuresis.

2. Bladder compliance following partial bladder outlet obstruction is diminished as a result of the following steps:

   (a) A rise in collagen mRNA, a rise in type I and III collagen, no change in tissue inhibitor of the matrix metalloproteinases (TIMP)
   (b) A rise in collagen mRNA, a rise in type I and III collagen, an increase in matrix metalloproteinase expression
   (c) Steady collagen mRNA, no change in type I and III collagen, no change in TIMP
   (d) A decline in collagen mRNA, a decline in type I and III collagen, increased matrix metalloproteinase expression
   (e) A rise in collagen mRNA, a rise in type I and III collagen, a rise in TIMP activity, and a decline in matrix metalloproteinase activity

   Answer: (e)   The deposition of large amounts of extracellular matrix elements affect the passive properties of the bladder wall and thus alter its storage characteristics. This increase in collagen protein expression is predominately of the types I and III, and is mediated by a rise in mRNA expression brought about by the impact of stretch on the bladder wall. This is accompanied by a loss of matrix metalloproteinase activity which is mediated by TIMP.

3. Which of the following statements best describes the use of fetal electrolytes to assess the renal prognosis:

   (a) Fetal electrolytes are highly predictive of future renal failure
   (b) The higher the osmolarity of the fetal urine, the better the renal prognosis
   (c) The best renal prognosis is seen if Na <100 meq/l, Cl <90 meq/l, and osmolarity is <210 mOsm/l
   (d) A single bladder aspiration is as reliable as multiple taps
   (e) The addition of β-2 microglobulin has supplanted fetal electrolytes as the marker of choice

   Answer: (c)   Severe fetal obstructive uropathy is associated with an isotonic urine. In contrast, a healthy fetal kidney will produce a very dilute urine. Despite nearly 25 years of clinical experience, fetal electrolytes still fail to fully predict renal failure. Up to one-third of patients with "favorable" fetal renal electrolytes still go on to develop renal insufficiency. Multiple bladder taps can increase the accuracy. The search for better markers with enhanced predictive power continues.

4. Fetal intervention for obstructive uropathy secondary to posterior urethral valves has been shown to:

    (a) Diminish the incidence of end-stage renal disease
    (b) Be associated with a high rate of fetal demise
    (c) Lead to improved pulmonary function in the neonate
    (d) Be most effective when accomplished by open fetal surgery
    (e) Be associated with neonatal respiratory failure

    Answer: (c)   Fetal intervention for posterior urethral valves has not been shown to lower the incidence of end-stage renal disease but, in properly selected cases, it can offer the benefit of improved neonatal pulmonary function. Neonates with severe obstructive uropathy die of respiratory failure due to a noncompliant and hypoplastic lung. While the fetal mortality has been reported to be high in older series with open procedures, fetal survival has improved with the less invasive method of fetal bladder shunting.

5. Which of the following clinical radiographic findings is not associated with an improved long-term renal prognosis?

    (a) Bilateral vesicoureteral reflux
    (b) Unilateral renal reflux into a dysplastic kidney
    (c) Bladder diverticulum

    (d) Urinary ascites
    (e) Perinephric urinoma

    Answer: (a)   All of the above findings except for bilateral vesicoureteral reflux are associated with a better long-term renal prognosis. These anatomic variants serve as pressure pop-off mechanisms and are associated with improved renal as well as bladder function.

6. A neonate presents following an antenatal diagnosis of severe bilateral hydroureteronephrosis. Postnatal imaging confirms a diagnosis of posterior urethral valves with a severely trabeculated bladder wall and bilateral vesicoureteral reflux. Despite an indwelling catheter, the neonate's creatinine rises to 3.1. There is a vigorous postobstructive diuresis noted and after 1 week the neonate is stable from a fluid and electrolytes standpoint, and the creatinine has settled at 2.6. Two days following a valve ablation, the creatinine rises again to 3.0 and a repeat ultrasound shows severe bilateral hydroureteronephrosis. Your best option for management is:

    (a) Repeat a voiding cystourethrography (VCUG) to search for a recurrent valve
    (b) Perform a vesicostomy
    (c) Institute clean intermittent catheterization (CIC)
    (d) Perform bilateral ureterostomies
    (e) Observation with serial sonograms

    Answer: (b)   This patient's clinical course is best explained by a smaller and noncompliant bladder coupled with a high urine output due to poor concentrating ability. This means that the entire system will reach a high and unfavorable storage pressure with a small amount of urinary volume, and because of the postobstructive diuresis, this volume will be reached in a short period of time. While some centers might advocate CIC in this setting, this means that the CIC would have to be performed at such frequent intervals as to become impractical. Furthermore, CIC in a patient with reflux carries the risk of developing a febrile urinary tract infection (UTI). Bilateral ureterostomies would lead to a defunctionalized bladder, which in this setting can aggravate the contracture process. Among these choices, we feel a vesicostomy is optimal because it will still allow for bladder cycling and yet prevent the high pressures from compromising both the bladder wall as well as the upper tracts.

7. A 3-year-old boy with a history of posterior urethral valves is transferred to your care with a fever of 104°F and a positive urine culture. He was maintained on bactrim prophylaxis and is noted to be uncircumcised. Sonography reveals a right kidney with moderate hydroureteronephrosis, and a left kidney with severe cortical atrophy and severe hydroureteronephrosis. A VCUG demonstrates unilateral high-grade reflux and a trabeculated bladder wall with no residual valve leaflets. The urine culture reveals *E. coli* sensitive to bactrim. Your management recommendation in this setting should be:

(a) Change the suppression antibiotic over to Keflex
(b) Start CIC
(c) Perform a circumcision
(d) Obtain a DMSA scan
(e) Perform a left nephroureterectomy

Answer: (c) Wiswell[2] was correct; prepuce presence portends the presence of perilous periurethral pathogens. While it is true that in normal males one must circumcise 99 boys to save 1 afebrile UTI, in the case of this toddler with severe posterior urethral valves, the stakes are much higher. Thus, in this instance, where it is likely that there was noncompliance with the prescribed medical course, a circumcision is reasonable. It is important to take a history

to understand why the bactrim prophylaxis failed, i.e. was it the taste of the antibiotic or an inability to pay for it. Even postcircumcision, this child should be maintained on prophylaxis. A DMSA scan will be less accurate in the setting of severe cortical atrophy. A left nephroureterectomy in this setting would mean that all of the urine output from the right kidney would be delivered to a bladder with less than optimal storage properties. Preserving the refluxing and nonfunctional left renal unit preserves compliance of the overall lower urinary tract and serves to protect the right kidney.

8. An 8-year-old boy presents with a history of posterior valves ablated in the neonatal period. He is proud to say that he is finally dry all day long and in underwear. But he is bothered by his nighttime wetting. His creatinine which was stable at 1.0 has now climbed to 1.5 and an ultrasound shows no significant change in the hydronephrosis seen over the years. Your next step should be:

(a) Praise him for being dry by day
(b) Tell his family that the creatinine goes up as boys get bigger
(c) Get a MAG3 renal scan to look for a kinking obstruction
(d) Get a uroflow with postvoid residual
(e) Have him keep a 72 voiding log with measured volumes and perform videourodynamics

Answer: (e) This boy will benefit from a videourodynamic study to assess his safe zone. The real question for this boy is at what volume does bladder pressure rise to a point which compromises renal function. Clinical and experimental studies have clearly shown that elevated bladder pressures are transmitted back to the renal pelves. Thus, as this young man seeks so desperately to be dry like his peers, he stresses his bladder by keeping it filled to the right side of the cystometry curve, which is in the zone of poor compliance. The key question is at what bladder volume is he out of his safe zone and this is best answered by a carefully done videourodynamic study. This study also will determine his postvoid residual urine. These data must then be correlated with his voiding log. In this manner his voiding habits can be restructured so as to keep his bladder working within its safe zone.

9. A 13-year-old boy presents for a videourodynamic study performed because of his persisting day and night wetting despite a successful neonatal valve ablation. A double lumen suprapubic catheter is inserted and 600 ml is drained. Fluoroscopic confirmation shows the bladder to be empty and bladder filling commences at 20 ml/min. At 35 min (700 ml) he reports the urge to void. He voids 500 ml with a slow stream and bilateral reflux is noted. The residual urine from the catheter is aspirated for and additional 500 ml with fluoroscopic confirmation to determine that both the bladder and upper tracts are contrast free. The optimal management for this boy is:

(a) Timed voiding
(b) CIC
(c) Overnight catheter drainage
(d) Timed voiding by day and overnight catheter drainage
(e) Bilateral reimplantation

Answer: (d) During their adolescent years it is not uncommon to see valve patients present with the syndrome of polyuria, urinary incontinence, and renal insufficiency. This subset of patients can be saved from end-stage renal disease if their bladder function is rigorously monitored and optimized. A valuable clue in this young man's case is that it took 700 ml for him to feel a need to void. For many of these boys, changes in the sensory innervation of the bladder have taken place such that they cannot even sense fullness until they are in the noncompliant danger zone of their cystometric curve. This young man voided with a slow stream but he carried a significant residual urine. For him timed voiding, and perhaps even double voiding by day, will work to keep him in the bladder's compliant safe zone. However, he has a significant postobstructive diuresis as manifested by the fact that while 700 ml of urine was instilled during the videourodynamic study, 1000 ml was voided or aspirated during the determination of the residual urine. What this means is that during a 35 min study, he made an additional 300 ml of urine, i.e. he had a postobstructive diuresis. In such an instance, overnight catheter drainage will preserve renal function and ultimately, in many instances, restore renal concentrating ability.

10. Which of the following statements is *not* true about the nature of postobstructive diuresis in the adolescent male with posterior urethral valves?

(a) They have decreased aquaporin expression in the ascending tubule
(b) They have noncompliant bladders
(c) They have diminished Cl- pump activity in the ascending loop of Henle
(d) The peak interstitial osmotic gradient within the medulla will be 800 mOsm/l
(e) There will be evidence of hypoxia within the medullary zone of the kidney

Answer: (d) A characteristic feature of boys with posterior valves is their diminished ability to concentrate urine. As infants they are thirstier than their peer group. As they grow older, parents often comment on the striking clarity of their urine. These boys will have a diminished interstitial medullary osmolarity; they will not have anything near the normal 800 mOsm/l gradient that serves to draw free water back in from the ascending tubule in the loop of Henle or the distal collecting ducts.

As the intrapelvic pressure remains elevated, substantial changes take place with diminished medullary blood flow which leads to hypoxia, which in turn contributes to a loss of the medullary concentration gradient. Decreased aquaporin expression as shown in experimental models of obstructive uropathy would also serve to increase the volume of dilute urine that is excreted.

References

1. Lapides J, Diokno AC, Silber SJ, Lowe BS. Clean, intermittent self-catheterization in the treatment of urinary tract disease. Trans Am Assoc Genitourin Surg 1971; 63: 92–6.
2. Wiswell TE, Miller GM, Gelston HM Jr, Jones SK, Clemmings AF. Effect of circumcision status on periurethral bacterial flora during the first year of life. J Pediatr 1988; 113: 442–6.

Prune belly syndrome

64

R Guy Hudson and Steven J Skoog

1. Prune belly syndrome is classically defined by all of the following abnormalities except:

   (a) Deficiency of the abdominal wall musculature
   (b) Hypospadias
   (c) Bilateral cryptorchidism
   (d) Dilated, dysmorphic urinary tract

   Answer: (b) Hypospadias is not a classic finding associated with prune belly syndrome.

2. Based on Woodard's classification, the majority of patients with prune belly syndrome reside in which category?

   (a) I
   (b) II
   (c) IIa
   (d) III
   (e) IV

   Answer: (d) Woodard described three major categories for children with prune belly syndrome, with Category III, the last category, to be the mildest. Category III patients are affected by the external abdominal features and undescended testes, but neither pulmonary nor renal function is significantly impaired.

3. The specific muscle layer most severely involved in prune belly syndrome is:

   (a) Transversus abdominis
   (b) Rectus abdominis below the umbilicus
   (c) Rectus abdominis above the umbilicus
   (d) Internal oblique
   (e) External oblique

   Answer: (a) The wrinkled, floppy abdominal wall which characterizes prune belly syndrome is due to a deficiency of the underlying musculature. The order of severity of involvement from most to least involved is: transversus abdominis; rectus abdominus below the umbilicus; internal oblique; and rectus abdominis above the umbilicus.

4. The most important/immediate factor which affects prognosis in the newborn with prune belly syndrome is:

   (a) Renal involvement
   (b) Pulmonary involvement
   (c) Cardiac involvement
   (d) Orthopedic abnormalities
   (e) Gastrointestinal abnormalities

   Answer: (a) Prognosis of a child with prune belly syndrome is directly related to renal function and the degree of renal dysplasia. It has been proposed that the renal dysplasia seen in prune belly syndrome is due to combination of a ureteric bud and metanephric defect.

5. All of the following are mandatory in the evaluation of a newborn with prune belly syndrome except:

   (a) Chest X-ray
   (b) Serum electrolytes
   (c) Urinalysis
   (d) Renal ultrasound
   (e) All of the above are mandatory in the initial evaluation of a newborn with prune belly syndrome

   Answer: (e) The neonatal evaluation in a child diagnosed with prune belly syndrome requires the physician to rule out pulmonary involvement, renal dysplasia and the presence of a urinary tract infection (UTI) among other factors.

6. Which of the following statements best describes the contour and capacity of the bladder in a patient with prune belly syndrome?

    (a) Thin walled, trabeculated, small capacity
    (b) Thick walled, trabeculated, small capacity
    (c) Thick walled, nontrabeculated, large capacity
    (d) Thin walled, trabeculated, large capacity
    (e) Thick walled, non-trabeculated, small capacity

    Answer: (c) The bladder in a child with prune belly syndrome is thick walled, enlarged, and nontrabeculated. The normal bladder contour is deviated by a pseudodiverticulum caused by the urachal remnant. The bladder neck is characteristically wide and vesicoureteral reflux is present.

7. The theory of mesodermal arrest as the etiology of prune belly syndrome fails to explain:

    (a) Absence of anatomic obstruction in most patients
    (b) Male predominance of the syndrome
    (c) High association with megalourethra
    (d) Abnormalities of the prostate and urethra
    (e) Abnormalities of testicular descent

    Answer: (b) The mesodermal arrest theory – that the abdominal wall and urinary tract would be vulnerable to a mesodermal defect occurring between 6 and 10 weeks of gestation – does not explain male predominance and the fact that abdominal wall abnormalities may be preset even with a normal urinary tract.

8. Which section of the ureter in patients with prune belly syndrome tends to be less

affected – an important consideration at the time of reconstructive surgery?

    (a) Proximal
    (b) Middle
    (c) Distal
    (d) Intramural
    (e) None of the above: all portions of the ureter are similarly affected in patients with prune belly syndrome

Answer: (a) The ureters are elongated, tortuous, and dilated in prune belly syndrome, and the lower third of the ureter is more affected than the proximal portion. True obstructive lesions of the ureter are rare.

9. All of the following can contribute to the etiology of infertility in patients with prune belly syndrome except:

    (a) Prostatic hypoplasia
    (b) Lack of continuity between the ductuli efferentes and rete testis
    (c) Abnormally thickened vas deferens and ectopic drainage
    (d) Atretic, absent or dilated seminal vesicles
    (e) All of the above can contribute to the etiology of infertility in patients with prune belly syndrome

Answer: (e) Infertility is strongly associated with prune belly syndrome and this is due to all of the anatomical factors described in choices (a)–(d). An open bladder neck and hypoplastic prostate result in retrograde ejaculation; abnormalities of the prostatic epithelium and seminal vesicles affect the seminal fluid; and vas deferens obstruction affects sperm delivery.

10. Undescended testes in patients with prune belly syndrome are usually located:

    (a) In the superficial inguinal pouch
    (b) In the inguinal canal
    (c) Intraabdominal, at the internal inguinal ring

(d) Intraabdominal, overlying the iliac vessels

(e) Intraabdominal, overlying the ecstatic ureters at the pelvic inlet

Answer: (e) Bilateral cryptorchidism is a hallmark of prune belly syndrome and the testes are usually in an intraabdominal portion overlying the ecstatic ureters at the pelvic inlet. The intraabdominal location of the testes is associated with the known risks of infertility and malignant degeneration.

11. The most common anterior urethral abnormality associated with patients with prune belly syndrome is:

(a) Megalourethra
(b) Hypospadias
(c) Microurethra
(d) Urethral duplication
(e) Nonobstructing bulbar urethral stricture

Answer: (a) The anterior urethral abnormalities associated with prune belly syndrome range from urethral atresia to fusiform megalourethra. Both scaphoid and fusiform megalourethra may be associated with prune belly syndrome.

12. The most frequent musculoskeletal/orthopedic abnormality in patients with prune belly syndrome is:

(a) Talipes equinovarus
(b) Polydactyly
(c) Congential dislocation of the hips
(d) Syndactyly
(e) Scoliosis

Answer: (c) Intrauterine compression and oligohydramnios may cause lateral dimples of the elbows and knees at the milder end of the spectrum, and, most commonly, congenital dislocation of the hips at the severe end. Scoliosis, talipes equinovarus, polydactyly and syndactyly are rare anomalies associated with prune belly syndrome.

Basic science of genitalia

65

CD Anthony Herndon
(Based on chapter written by Laurence S Baskin)

1. The critical gene responsible for male sexual differentiation is:

   (a) LIM-1
   (b) SOX-9
   (c) SRY
   (d) DAX-1
   (e) WT-1

   Answer: (c) Products of the SRY gene located on the short arm of chromosome Y initiate the cascade of events which leads to male differentiation via development of the testis.

2. Germ cells are derived from which layer:

   (a) Ectoderm
   (b) Mesoderm
   (c) Endoderm
   (d) None of the above

   Answer: (c) Germs cells are derived from the endoderm cell layer.

3. The critical gene responsible for female sexual differentiation is:

   (a) LIM-1
   (b) SOX-9
   (c) SRY
   (d) DAX-1
   (e) WT-1

   Answer: (d) Once thought to be the default pathway, the DAX-1 gene located on the X chromosome is felt to be critical in the pathway of female sexual development. The DAX-1 gene does not appear to be active when present with the SRY gene and the Y chromosome.

4. In the presence of the SRY gene, which compound facilitates the conversions of cholesterol to pregnenolone?

   (a) 11-B hydroxylase
   (b) 5-alpha reductace
   (c) Steroidogenesis acute regulatory (STAR) protein
   (d) 21-alpha hydroxylase
   (e) 19-aromatase

   Answer: (c) In the normal male, SRY overwhelms the DAX-1 gene resulting in the STAR protein being the first step in steroidogenesis facilitating the conversion of cholesterol to pregnenolone.

5. Which protein induces the regression of the Müllerian ducts?

   (a) Free testosterone
   (b) DHT
   (c) MIS
   (d) SRY
   (e) STAR protein

   Answer: (c) MIS produced from the Sertoli cells directly inhibits formation of the Müllerian duct system. This acts locally and lateralizes to the affected side.

6. Which structures are not derived from the Müllerian duct system?

(a) Upper one-fifth of vagina
(b) Fallopian tube
(c) Uterus
(d) Cervix
(e) Clitoris

Answer: (e) The clitoris is derived from the genital tubercle. All other structures are derived from the Müllerian duct system. The urethra and lower vagina are derived from the urinogenital sinus and urethral folds.

Basic science of the testis — 66

Stephen Lukasewycz and Aseem R Shukla

(Based on chapter written by Julia Spencer Barthold)

1. Regarding gonadal determination, which of the following statements is false?

   (a) In the human fetus, formation of the indifferent gonadal ridge occurs at 33 days
   (b) Expression of WT1, though possibly associated with murine gonadal determination, has not yet been determined to play a role in human gonadal development
   (c) Mutations in SF1, a transcription factor, are associated with XY gonadal dysgenesis in humans
   (d) SF1 interacts with many other transcription factors including Sry, Sox9, and AMH in its role in gonadal determination
   (e) All of the above are true

   Answer: (b) The indifferent gondal ridge does begin to form at 33 days gestation. Mutations in SFI have been associated with XY gonadal dysgenesis but not with failure of ovarian or adrenal development. SF1 does interact with numerous downstream factors. Answer (b) is false because WT1 is a transcription factor required for normal development of the urogenital ridge and for germ cell development in both mice and men.

2. All of the following are true except:

   (a) The SRY gene is involved with gonadal development and not gonadal determination
   (b) Pre-Leydig cells begin expressing SRY at 41 days gestation
   (c) SRY is the sex-determining region on the Y choromosome
   (d) WT1 and SF1 are the two genes known to be required for gonadal determination and not development
   (e) All of the above are true

   Answer: (b) Pre-Sertoli cells begin expressing SRY at 41 days gestation; Leydig cells do not express SRY. The remainder of the choices above are true.

3. What percentage of individuals with XY gonadal dysgenesis have mutations of SRY?

   (a) 5–10%
   (b) 15–20%
   (c) 25–30%
   (d) 35–40%
   (e) 50–65%

   Answer: (b) Although SRY is critical in testis development, only 15–20% of individuals with XY dysgenesis have mutations of SRY. Other genetic and environmental factors are likely the cause in other individuals with XY dysgenesis.

4. Regarding Amh and AMH (anti-Müllerian hormone) which of the following are false?

   (a) Amh is a member of the transforming growth factor-β family
   (b) Secretion of AMH is inhibited by Wnt4 and Dax1 in the ovary

(c) Males with a deletion of Amh have persistence of Müllerian structures but have normal fertility

(d) AMH is a sensitive indicator of the function of Sertoli cells

(e) All of the above are true

Answer: (c)   AMH is a member of the transforming growth factor-β family and is a sensitive measure of Sertoli cell function. AMH is inhibited by Wnt4 and Dax1 in the ovary. Clinically, males with a deletion of Amh have persistence of Müllerian structures, and also have testicular dysgenesis and infertility.

5. All of the below are true regarding the role of INSL3 in testicular descent except?

(a) Insl3 is a G-protein coupled receptor on the gubernaculum thought to stimulate gubernacular growth when bound by G-protein coupled receptor affecting testicular descent (GREAT)

(b) The majority of infants with isolated cryptorchidism will demonstrate a mutation in INSL3

(c) INSL3 is a hormone in the relaxin family that is a nonandrogenic testicular factor

(d) Homozygous deletion of Insl3 and Rxfp2 in mice is associated with perirenal testes and failure of gubernacular development

(e) All of the above are true

Answer: (b)   Insl 3 and the GREAT were expected to be candidate genes for human nonsyndromic cryptorchidism, but a mutation in one of these genes is present in <5% of cases. A multifactorial etiology involving several genes and external exposures is likely responsible.

Hsi-Yang Wu and Howard M Snyder III

1. A patient who is a true hermaphrodite is found on gonadal biopsy to have a right ovotestis and a left ovary. Which arrangement of the internal genital anatomy would cause you to question the adequacy of the gonadal biopsy?

   (a) Bilateral fallopian tubes
   (b) Right fallopian tube, left fallopian tube and vas
   (c) Right fallopian tube and vas, left fallopian tube
   (d) Right fallopian tube, left fallopian tube with atretic hemiuterus
   (e) Right fallopian tube, left fallopian tube with normal hemiuterus

   Answer: (b)   The internal structures ipsilateral to an ovotestis can be either a fallopian tube or a fallopian tube and vas. However, a vas cannot be found ipsilateral to an ovary. If a patient has an ovotestis in which the testicular portion is deep to the ovarian portion, then it is possible to miss the deeper portion with a superficial gonadal biopsy.

2. A newborn is noted to have no palpable gonads, moderate phallic enlargement and fusion of the labial/scrotal folds with a urethral meatus at the base of the phallus. The lab test most likely to indicate the correct diagnosis is:

   (a) 17-hydroxyprogesterone
   (b) Corticosterone
   (c) Cortisol
   (d) Testosterone
   (e) Dihydrotestosterone (DHT)

   Answer: (a)   By physical exam, this patient is most likely a female due to a lack of palpable gonads and the likely diagnosis is congenital adrenal hyperplasia (CAH). If a male pseudohermaphrodite had this physical exam, then the testosterone and DHT levels could be elevated or low. Finding an elevated 17-hydroxyprogesterone level would rule out any of the male pseudohermaphrodite conditions.

3. You are seeing as 8-year-old patient, who is a recent immigrant, for ambiguous genitalia, and who has other relatives with ambiguous genitalia. The left gonad is descended and the right one is at the pubic tubercle. The urethra has a perineal opening and the phallus is small. Which lab test will allow you to determine the diagnosis without performing a gonadal biopsy?

   (a) 17-hydroxyprogesterone
   (b) Cortisol
   (c) Testosterone/DHT ratio
   (d) Dihydroepiandrosterone
   (e) Luteinizing hormone (LH), follicle-stimulating hormone (FSH)

   Answer: (c)   The patient is a male pseudohermaphrodite, most likely with 5α-reductase deficiency. A testosterone/DHT ratio of 50:1 will confirm the diagnosis.

4. Which intersex patient is potentially fertile?

  (a) Partial androgen insensitivity
  (b) True hermaphrodite, female sex of rearing
  (c) Gonadal dysgenesis, 46,XY karyotype
  (d) Mixed gonadal dysgenesis
  (e) 20,22 desmolase (StAR protein) deficiency

  Answer: (b)   From this group, only true hermaphrodites with a female sex of rearing have a chance of being fertile (Table 68.1). True hermaphrodites with a male sex of rearing have abnormal testicular function which makes fertility rare. The only intersex patients who have normal fertility potential are those with CAH.

5. In which intersex state is there no increased risk of gonadal malignancy?

  (a) Persistent Müllerian duct syndrome
  (b) Gonadal dysgenesis, 46,XX karyotype
  (c) Mixed gonadal dysgenesis
  (d) True hermaphrodite, male sex of rearing
  (e) Complete androgen insensitivity

  Answer: (b)   The presence of a Y chromosome and an undescended testis increases the risk of gonadal malignancy; therefore, the patient with a 46,XX karyotype is not at increased risk.

6. A phenotypic male presents with a nonpalpable right testis and a large left inguinal hernia. The left hernia sac is found to contain a uterus, fallopian tubes, and a gonad that looks like a testis. This condition is due to a defect in:

  (a) 20,22 desmolase (StAR protein)
  (b) 3β-hydroxysteroid dehydrogenase (HSD3B2)
  (c) 21-hydroxylase (CYP21)

  (d) Müllerian-inhibiting substance
  (e) 5α-reductase

  Answer: (d)   This is the classic presentation of persistent Müllerian duct syndrome, a male who is discovered on inguinal exploration to have female internal gonadal structures. Patients with StAR protein deficiency are phenotypically female and the remainder have ambiguous genitalia rather than appearing male.

7. A phenotypic female presents at 1 year of age with a left inguinal hernia. The sac contains a gonad without an associated fallopian tube. The diagnosis can be established by all except:

  (a) Rectal exam to palpate cervix
  (b) Pelvic ultrasound
  (c) Vaginoscopy
  (d) 17-hydroxyprogesterone
  (e) Magnetic resonance imaging (MRI) of pelvis

  Answer: (d)   The concern is whether this child has unrecognized complete androgen insensitivity syndrome. The presence of a uterus can be determined by (a), (b), (c) or (e). Without clitoral hypertrophy, it is unlikely that 17-hydroxyprogesterone will be elevated.

8. You are discussing prenatal treatment with a family whose previous girls have been affected with CAH. As you discuss the risks and benefits of treatment, what is the likelihood that prenatal steroid treatment will prevent masculinization of the fetus?

  (a) 100%, it is an autosomal dominant condition
  (b) 50%, it is autosomal dominant but only females would benefit
  (c) 25%, it is an autosomal recessive condition

(d) 12.5%, it is an autosomal recessive condition but only females would benefit

(e) Unknown, it is a random mutation

Answer: (d) Only females would benefit from treatment of this autosomal recessive condition. (Page 1153).

9. Patients with CAH may be hypertensive because:

(a) 17-hydroxyprogesterone, a strong glucocorticoid is elevated in 21-hydroxylase deficiency

(b) Dihydroepiandrosterone, a sex steroid is elevated in 3β-hydroxysteroid dehydrogenase deficiency

(c) Progesterone affects renal vascular resistance

(d) Cholesterol distention of the adrenal causes excess renin release

(e) Deoxycorticosterone, a strong mineralocorticoid is elevated in 11α-hydroxlase deficiency

Answer: (e) Excess mineralocorticoid causes hypertension. Most patients with CAH require replacement of mineralocorticoid and may present with shock. (c) and (d) are not physiological mechanisms.

10. During performance of a right gonadectomy and hypospadias repair on a boy with mixed gonadal dysgenesis and 45,XO/46,XY karyotype, a small hemiuterus is encountered and removed. The left testis is descended in the scrotum. Why did this child have a hemiuterus?

(a) He has undiagnosed persistent Müllerian duct syndrome and has a hemiuterus on the left as well

(b) The streak gonad did not express Müllerian inhibiting substance (MIS), therefore the uterus did not involute

(c) He has low 5α-reductase levels

(d) He is an undiagnosed true hermaphrodite

(e) He has undiagnosed pure gonadal dysgenesis

Answer: (b) Although the presence of the hemiuterus is due to the lack of MIS, it affects only the side ipsilateral to the streak gonad. He has normal Wolffian structures on the left side. DHT affects only external genital development. The karyotype rules out true hermaphroditism or pure gonadal dysgenesis.

Imperforate anus and cloaca

Curtis Sheldon and William R DeFoor Jr

1. All of the following clinical characteristics suggest a "high" level imperforate anus which will likely require a neonatal diverting colostomy except:

   (a) Meconium passage from the urethra or bladder
   (b) "Rocker-bottom" perineum
   (c) Perineal fistula
   (d) Rectovaginal or rectovestibular fistula
   (e) Radiographically determined distance between the rectal pouch and perineum exceeding 1 cm

   Answer: (c) The presence of a perineal fistula generally denotes a "low" level lesion that may be amenable to a neonatal posterior sagittal anorectoplasty and thus avoid a diverting colostomy.

2. Neonatal management of patients with anorectal malformations includes all of the following except:

   (a) Normalization of anorectal anatomy
   (b) Protect the upper urinary tracts from obstruction and stasis
   (c) Ensure low-pressure bladder drainage
   (d) Minimize any neurologic deficit that might arise from treatable spinal pathology
   (e) Achieve fecal continence

   Answer: (e) Neonatal management of anorectal malformations includes minimizing complications to the genitourinary system and assessing for associated neurological conditions. Fecal continence is addressed around the age of toilet training with bowel management.

3. *Initial* neonatal urologic evaluation includes all of the following except:

   (a) Renal and bladder ultrasound
   (b) Filling cystometrogram
   (c) Voiding cystourethrogram
   (d) Postvoid residual
   (e) Spinal ultrasound

   Answer: (b) A thorough anatomical evaluation of the urinary tract and spine is essential in the newborn period to assess for associated anomalies. A urodynamics study can be helpful in diagnosing and following a neuropathic bladder but is difficult to interpret in the newborn and is not critical to the initial evaluation.

4. Severe bladder dysfunction diagnosed in the neonatal period may require which of the following:

   (a) Clean intermittent catheterization
   (b) Cutaneous vesicostomy
   (c) Anticholinergic medication
   (d) Antibiotic prophylaxis
   (e) All of the above

   Answer: (e) High bladder pressures with incomplete emptying and/or detrusor–external sphincter dyssynergia may lead to urinary stasis, vesicoureteral reflux, and upper tract injury. Urologic intervention is indicated when a neuropathic bladder is suspected and is more common with "high" anorectal malformation lesions.

5. The following type of fecal diversion is preferred in patients with a high anorectal malformation:

   (a) Transverse
   (b) Descending loop
   (c) Descending with completely separated stomas
   (d) Ascending
   (e) Ileostomy

   Answer: (c)   A colostomy performed at the junction of the descending and sigmoid colon with separated stomas is preferable to prevent fecal contamination of the urinary tract and completely decompress the distal colon.

6. Metabolic complications of urine passing from the bladder, through a rectovesical or rectourethral fistula and into the defunctionalized distal limb of colon following initial diverting colostomy includes the following:

   (a) Hypernatremia
   (b) Metabolic alkalosis
   (c) Hyponatremia
   (d) Hyperchloremic metabolic acidosis
   (e) Hyperkalemia

   Answer: (d)   This condition usually occurs as the result of urine passing from the bladder, through a rectovesical or rectourethral fistula and into the defunctionalized distal limb of colon following initial diverting colostomy. The resultant absorption of urinary constituents by the bowel results in the metabolic abnormality. The occurrence of this complication requires the presence of a urorectal fistula and is facilitated by a long segment of defunctionalized colon (large absorptive surface) communicating with the fistula. Additionally, the presence of distal urinary obstruction, which may be structural (stricture) or functional (neurovesical dysfunction), facilitates this risk. Urinary tract infection and renal insufficiency may also exacerbate this metabolic abnormality. Hyperchloremic metabolic acidosis may be avoided by the creation of a low, fully diverting colostomy and by ensuring effective bladder drainage.

7. The level of the rectal insertion in a female with a persistent cloaca should be clinically or radiographically determined in the initial neonatal assessment. True or false?

   Answer: False   From a surgical perspective, the level of insertion of the rectum is generally immaterial, as all patients are managed with an initial diverting colostomy. The presence of a cloacal malformation is an urgent indication for the creation of a colostomy in order to prevent fecal contamination of the urinary tract. The colostomy should be positioned so as to be well away from the lower midline abdomen, where a subsequent vesicostomy may be necessary.

8. Initial management of a patient with a persistent cloaca includes all of the following except:

   (a) Diverting colostomy
   (b) Drainage of hydrocolpos
   (c) Genitourinary evaluation
   (d) Spinal evaluation
   (e) Posterior sagittal anorectal urethrovaginoplasty (PSARUVP)

   Answer: (e)   During the first phase of management, attention is directed towards protection of the upper urinary tracts, the maintenance of low-pressure urinary drainage, normalization of perineal anatomy, and minimalization of any neurologic deficit related to spinal cord anomaly. The presence of a cloacal malformation is an urgent indication for the creation of a colostomy in order to prevent fecal contamination of the urinary tract. The definitive repair of the cloacal malformation is deferred until 3–6 months of age after a careful endoscopic assessment of the common channel and a thorough bowel preparation.

9. Long-term follow-up of cloacal patients includes periodic gynecological assessments as well as colorectal and urological evaluations. True or false?

    Answer: True   Long-term gynecologic problems have been reported after cloacal reconstruction. A significant number of patients have reached adolescence and suffered from hematometra or hematocolpos. Recommendations have been made to detect atresias of the Müllerian system early in life and reassess these patients at early puberty by imaging and perhaps vaginoscopy.

10. Patients with a cloaca should never have their anorectal and urogenital sinus malformations corrected separately. True or false?

    Answer: True   The best results are attained by a single-stage PSARUVP. Those patients who present for correction of a urogenital sinus malformation who have previously undergone an anorectal pull-through procedure are best corrected by reoperative PSAR-UVP complete with repeat mobilization of the rectum.

1. In regards to genital development, which of the following statements is correct?

   (a) The vagina has two embryologic components, the paramesonephric ducts, and sinovaginal bulb

   (b) The secretion of Müllerian-inhibiting substance (MIS) from the Leydig cells causes the mesonephric ducts to involute

   (c) The paramesonephric ducts give rise to the epididymis, vas deferens, and seminal vesicles

   (d) Under the influence of the H-Y gene the bipotential gonad should differentiate into an ovary around 7 weeks gestation

   (e) Embryologic errors in the urogenital tract have a relatively narrow spectrum of severity

   Answer: (a)   Under the influence of SRY (the sex-determining region of the Y chromosome) the bipotential gonad differentiates into a testis near the 7th week of gestation. Normal phenotypic expression of male differentiation is actively controlled by secretion of MIS by Sertoli cells and testosterone by Leydig cells. MIS causes regression of the paramesonephric (Müllerian) ducts between 8 and 10 weeks of gestation. In females, the absence of the Y chromosome and SRY protein secretion leads to the formation of ovaries. Without MIS and androgen secretion, the paramesonephric ducts give rise to the fallopian tubes, uterus, and the upper two-thirds of the vagina. The distal third of the vagina is formed from the sinovaginal bulb.

2. A patient with a urogenital sinus abnormality ____:

   (a) Exhibits a common channel into which the urethra, vagina, and rectum empty

   (b) Commonly has associated abnormalities of the clitoris, labia, and external genitalia

   (c) Will most likely have pure gonadal dysgenesis as their medical diagnosis

   (d) Should undergo a thorough medical evaluation electively as an outpatient at 1–2 months of age

   (e) Requires only renal ultrasound during radiographic evaluation

   Answer: (b)   A urogenital sinus abnormality is present when the urethra and vagina are joined and exit the perineum as a common channel. A persistent cloaca or cloacal anomaly exists when a single perineal opening drains the bladder, vagina, and rectum. Patients with urogenital sinus anomalies commonly have abnormalities of the clitoris, labia, and external genitalia. A thorough medical evaluation of the newborn with a urogenital sinus should be completed as many of these children will have congenital adrenal hyperplasia (CAH). Delays in diagnosis can lead to life-threatening fluid and electrolyte abnormalities. In addition to abdominal and pelvic sonography, all patients should undergo contrast genitography to help define the length of the common sinus and the level of confluence.

3. Which of the following statements is correct regarding current surgical techniques for clitoroplasty?

   (a) They are typically performed in the adolescent period
   (b) A dorsal tunical incision is made in the hope of preserving clitoral nerve supply
   (c) Clitoral amputation is a reasonable surgical alternative
   (d) Subtunical resection of the corpora may preserve glanular blood supply
   (e) Erectile tissue should only be excised in patients with massive clitoral enlargement

Answer: (d) Current clitoroplasty techniques are based on Schmid's description of corporal body excision and neurovascular bundle conservation. Subtunical resection of the corporal erectile tissue with preservation of the dorsal tunica may protect the glanular nerve and blood supply.[1] Baskin and colleagues have suggested that a more ventral tunical incision may be prudent after carefully demonstrating lateral fanning of the clitoral nerve supply.[2] Erectile tissue is routinely excised from the proximal bifurcation out to the level of the corona along with the ventral tunics. Clitoral reduction is typically performed within the first year of life. Early intervention may carry the benefit of thicker, more vascular skin and easier dissection of the clitoris and paravaginal tissue related to maternal estrogen stimulation.

4. In patients with a low vaginal confluence which of the following statements is correct?

   (a) Cutback vaginoplasty is a common and highly successful method of treatment
   (b) The flap should be V-shaped to avoid distortion of the perineum
   (c) During flap vaginoplasty a broad-based perineal flap is advanced into the incised vagina posteriorly

   (d) The use of the flap vaginoplasty easily corrects the urogenital sinus abnormality during flap mobilization and tailoring
   (e) The cutback vaginoplasty technique involves complicated flap harvesting and subsequent tissue modeling

Answer: (c) A cutback vaginoplasty is performed in the patient with labial fusion and is rarely indicated. This simple procedure involves making an incision in the fused skin posteriorly to the perineum and then oversewing the incised lateral edges. Flap vaginoplasty is best suited for those patients with a low confluence of the urogenital sinus. Maintaining a U rather than narrow V shape at the tip helps maintain vascularity. Modification of the distal flap into a rhomboid or omega shape allows for subsequent use of the labia to provide posterior closure of the introitus. Flap vaginoplasty does not correct the urogenital sinus. Without any separation of the vagina from urethra, the patient is still left with a urogenital sinus.

5. Surgical correction of the patient with a high vaginal confluence using the pull-through vaginoplasty technique ____:

   (a) Involves relatively easy tissue dissection and separation
   (b) Had early results which produced an isolated and anteriorly displaced urethra
   (c) Has had several recent modifications to improve surgical exposure
   (d) Had rare problems related to vaginal stenosis following aggressive mobilization of the vagina
   (e) Places the patient at particular risk for the development of a urethrovaginal fistula at the most distal aspect of the repair

Answer: (c) The pull-through vaginoplasty technique is a challenging procedure as establishing the proper plane between the proximal urethra and anterior urethra is very difficult.

Early results produced an unappealing, isolated and separate vaginal opening. Vaginal stenosis has been reported and is likely due to tension created by attempts to mobilize the relatively thin vagina all the way to the perineum. Most urethrovaginal fistulae occur at the level of the initial confluence where the exposure and repair are most tenuous. Modifications of this technique to improve exposure include the transtrigonal, posterior sagittal, and anterior sagittal approach.[3–5]

6. The technique of total urogenital mobilization _____ :

    (a) Is used extensively in patients with a low vaginal confluence
    (b) Has been shown by several well-designed studies to cause transient urinary and fecal incontinence, which improves with pelvic floor exercises
    (c) Has revolutionized the treatment of patients with high vaginal confluences
    (d) Is best suited for those patients with a mid-level confluence, allowing for subsequent flap vaginoplasty following mobilization
    (e) Is performed solely in the low lithotomy position

Answer: (d)   Urogenital mobilization is generally not necessary for patients with a low confluence. The best indication for its use may be patients with a mid-level lesion in whom the level of confluence may be converted to a low one suitable for flap vaginoplasty. The role of total urogenital mobilization for patients with a high level confluence remains to be determined. A full, lower body surgical prep from the nipple to toes, front to back, allows exposure to the entire lower body in both the prone and supine position, which may be required for exposure. Quality reviews documenting long-term results following feminizing genitoplasty or vaginoplasty in the setting of a urogenital sinus are lacking.

7. Which of the following statements is correct regarding vaginal replacement?

    (a) Bowel vaginoplasty has as its advantages, natural lubrication and less frequent issues with contracture of the neovagina
    (b) Chronic vaginal dilatation of the perineum typically provides an accommodating vagina with few problems related to dyspareunia
    (c) Split-thickness skin grafts have minor problems with graft contracture and rarely require chronic vaginal dilatation
    (d) The preferred bowel segment used during the creation of a bowel neovagina is the transverse colon
    (e) Full-thickness skin grafts provide substantially more lubrication than split-thickness skin grafts and are preferred for vaginal replacement

Answer: (a)   Advantages of bowel vaginoplasty include natural lubrication from the intestinal segment, fewer problems with dyspareunia, and infrequent contracture or stenosis, usually without any need for routine vaginal dilatation. Sigmoid colon or ileum are the preferred segments for the creation of a neovagina because of their proximity and ease of mobility of these bowel segments into the pelvis. Full-thickness skin grafts have less reliable ingrowth of blood supply but contract less once in place in comparison to split-thickness skin grafts. Chronic vaginal dilatation of the perineum does not create an adequate vagina and leads to dyspareunia.

8. Long-term results following genital reconstruction demonstrate _____ :

    (a) Normal orgasm and sexual satisfaction in almost all patients
    (b) Rare problems associated with vaginal stenosis using older, time-tested methods
    (c) That all patients undergoing vaginoplasty would benefit from the total urogenital mobilization technique

(d) That novel laparoscopic approaches are helpful with dissection and separation of the proximal vagina and urethra

(e) The need for an improved analysis of all patients in regards to urinary and sexual function, and quality of life issues

Answer: (e) Quality reviews documenting long-term results following feminizing genitoplasty or vaginoplasty in the setting of a urogenital sinus are lacking, particularly any study with careful consideration of the initial anatomy or the surgical technique employed. A number of studies have evaluated the vagina after reconstruction in terms of vaginal stenosis and these reviews reported high rates (>30%) of secondary procedures performed to correct stenosis. Total urogenital mobilization is most helpful in patients with mid-level lesions providing improved exposure and potentially easier dissection leading to decreased operative time, and possibly fewer complications. Laparoscopy is not a technique currently employed to help in the dissection or exposure of the urogenital sinus during reconstruction.

References

1. Kogan SJ, Smey P, Levitt SB. Subtunical total reduction clitoroplasty: a safe modification of existing techniques. J Urol 1983; 130: 746–8.
2. Baskin LS, Erol A, Li YW et al. Anatomical studies of the human clitoris. J Urol 1999; 162: 1015–20.
3. Passerini-Glazel G. A new 1 stage procedure for clitorovaginoplasty in severely masculinized female pseudohermaphrodites. J Urol 1989; 142: 565–8.
4. Pena A, Filmer B, Bonilla E, Mendez M, Stolar C. Transanorectal approach for the treatment of the urogenital sinus: preliminary report. J Pediatr Surg 1992; 27: 681–5.
5. Rink RC, Pope JC, Kropp BP et al. Reconstruction of the high urogenital sinus: early perineal prone approach without division of the rectum. J Urol 1997; 158: 1293–7.

Hypospadias

71

Warren T Snodgrass, Aseem R Shukla, and Douglas A Canning

1. A boy presents 5 years after distal hypospadias repair complaining of a slow stream and straining to void. On physical examination a faint white line is seen along the margins of a small-appearing meatus. He voided 170 ml with a peak flow of 4 ml/s and a plateau-shaped curve. Intervention most likely to correct this problem is:

   (a) Meatal dilation
   (b) Meatotomy
   (c) Reoperative urethroplasty using a flip-flap from the ventral skin
   (d) Single-stage reoperation using a buccal inlay graft
   (e) Two-stage buccal graft urethroplasty

   Answer: (e)   Late presentation of obstructive symptoms and white discoloration at the meatus suggest balantis xerotica obliterans (BXO). While any of the mentioned therapies might have short-term success, control of BXO requires all involved tissues be excised. The resultant defect is best corrected using a staged buccal graft, since graft-take is more reliable in reoperations with a staged approach and BXO recurs in genital and nongenital skin, but has not yet been reported in buccal mucosa. Intraoperative biopsy for frozen section has in our experience not been feasible to obtain sufficient tissue for diagnosis while preserving enough tissue for single-stage repair if results are negative.

2. The main contraindication to primary tubularized incised plate (TIP) urethroplasty is:

   (a) Proximal hypospadias
   (b) A narrow urethral plate
   (c) Ventral curvature >45° after the penis is degloved
   (d) Repair in adults
   (e) A flat urethral plate with minimal glans groove

   Answer: (c)   There is no apparent glans–urethral plate configuration (i.e. a narrow versus wide plate or a flat versus deeply grooved plate) which prevents TIP repair. Similarly, it potentially can be used for any extent of hypospadias. The main contraindication is significant ventral curvature persisting after the penis is degloved, which leads to transection of the plate for straightening.

3. All of the following are thought to reduce likelihood of fistulas in distal hypospadias repair except:

   (a) Taking care not to tubularize the neourethra too far distally
   (b) Two-layer closure of the neourethra
   (c) Subepithelial stitching of the neourethra
   (d) Covering the neourethra with a dartos flap
   (e) Using a urethral stent postoperatively

   Answer: (e)   Urinary diversion with a urethral catheter has been a source of controversy in primary hypospadias repair, especially for distal hypospadias. There is no clear evidence that catheters reduce the fistula rate in distal operations. Also, reoperations to close small fistulas can be done successfully without catheters.

4. While a definite etiology for hypospadias remains elusive, all of the following are considered contributing factors except:

    (a) Abnormal androgen production by the fetal testis
    (b) Mutation at the Great/Lgr8 gene causing lack of binding at the insulin-3 receptor
    (c) Limited androgen sensitivity in target tissues of the developing genitalia
    (d) Premature loss of androgenic stimulation due to early atrophy of Leydig cells of the testis

    Answer: (b) The Great/Lgr8 gene regulates the receptor for insulin-3, a hormone which is a primary stimulus to gubernacular growth. All of the other listed factors are felt to contribute to the incomplete embryologic development which results in hypospadias.

5. The urethral plate, corpus spongiosum, and corpora cavernosa are derived from the:

    (a) Endoderm
    (b) Mesoderm
    (c) Ectoderm
    (d) Genital swelling
    (e) Coronal sulcus

    Answer: (b) Androgen stimulation causes the genital tubercle to elongate and the urogenital folds to migrate toward the midline and fuse moving proximally to distally. As the plate tubularizes, mesoderm within the urethral folds differentiates into the urethral plate and corporal bodies.

6. Chordee, or ventral penile curvature, often associated with hypospadias, is now believed to be the result of:

    (a) Fibrous bands attaching along the ventral half of the penis along the corpora cavernosa and reaching into the intercorporeal septum
    (b) A dysgenetic urethral plate which tethers the glans of the penis causing ventral tilting
    (c) Poorly vascularized subepithelial tissue dorsal to the urethral plate
    (d) Ventral corporeal disproportion
    (e) Persistence of embryologic ventral bow-strings which bridge between glans and the penoscrotal junction

    Answer: (d) While early surgeons believed that excision of "fibrous bands" at the ventrum of the penis was required to straighten the penis, chordee is now believed to be caused by ventral corporeal disproportion. Either the Nesbit dorsal plication or incision and corporeal grafting are now utilized to correct corporal disproportion. Subepithelial biopsies of the urethral plate revealed only well-vascularized connective tissues without fibrosis.

7. The TIP urethroplasty and onlay island flap hypospadias repairs share all of the following except:

    (a) Both repairs rely upon local urethral tissue for the reconstruction of the neourethra
    (b) Both repairs may be used for both proximal and distal repairs as long as the chordee can be corrected without transecting the urethral plate
    (c) Properly completed, the TIP and island onlay result share a low risk of fistula and meatal stenosis
    (d) Incising the distal urethral plate during an island onlay repair, before the glansplasty, results in a slit-like urethral meatus as is obtained after a TIP repair

(e) Subcuticular suture placement seems to improve cosmesis and decrease the fistula rate for both types of repairs

Answer: (a)   The onlay island flap hypospadias repair is based on the inner prepuce, transposed ventrally on a pudendal arterial supplied dartos mesentery skin flap that is overlaid on the urethral plate. The TIP repair depends on the intrinsic urethral plate but may be buttressed by the dartos mesentery transposed ventrally to cover the suture line.

8. The most important technical step to avoid turbulent voiding, kinking, and diverticulum formation after an onlay island flap is to:

(a) Leave redundancy in the island flap epithelium to avoid the possibility of stricture formation
(b) Aggressively trim the proximal flap to a wedge shape to provide a consistent caliber of the tube as the neourethra meets the native urethra
(c) Measure the combined width of the preserved urethral plate and flap to be about 20 mm, and no wider at the anastomosis than at the urethral urethral meatus
(d) Incorporate the neourethra with every stitch of a glansplasty
(e) Remove excess dorsal preputial skin as it is unlikely to be viable for use in circumferential skin coverage

Answer: (b)   The key step in preventing the complications of a diverticulum and turbulent voiding is to aggressively trim the flap proximally to a wedge shape, and overall so that the combined width of the plate and flap is no more than 10 mm. The neourethra may be incorporated in the first stitch of a glansplasty and excess dorsal preputial skin is split in the midline and rotated ventrally to afford adequate skin coverage in a typical hypospadias repair.

Abnormalities of the penis and scrotum

72

Stephen Lukasewycz and Aseem R Shukla

(Based on chapter written by Michael MacDonald, Julie Spencer Barthold, and Evan J Kass)

1. What percentage of males age 11–15 should be able to completely retract their prepuce?

   (a) 96%
   (b) 86%
   (c) 76%
   (d) 66%
   (e) 56%

   Answer: (d) Over time the physiologic adherence between the glans and inner preputial skin decreases. By age 11–15 two-thirds of boys are able to retract their foreskin completely and 95% of boys aged 16–17 can completely retract their foreskin.

2. Which of the following statements regarding meatal stenosis is true (select all that apply):

   (a) Meatal stenosis occurs in both circumcised and uncircumcised boys with equal frequency
   (b) Frenular devascularization during circumcision is one proposed etiology of meatal stenosis
   (c) Upward deflection of the urinary stream is most often caused by high-pressure voiding of childhood and is not often associated with meatal stenosis
   (d) Chronic meatitis from exposure to urine in the diaper is one proposed etiology of meatal stenosis

   Answer: (b), (d) Meatal stenosis occurs almost exclusively in circumcised males. Proposed mechanisms include frenular artery devascularization and chronic meatitis. An upward deflection of the urinary stream is pathognomonic.

3. A newborn male is noted to have a stretched penile length of 1.5 cm. Work-up should include:

   (a) Karyotype
   (b) Alpha fetoprotein (AFP)
   (c) No work-up is necessary, penis length is within normal limits
   (d) Inhibin level
   (e) No work-up is necessary, but treatment should include intramuscular (IM) testosterone

   Answer: (a) Micropenis by definition is 2–2.5 standard deviations below the mean for age. For a newborn penis, a stretched length of <2.0 cm fits this criteria. Work-up should evaluate for gonadotropin deficiency and testicular dysgenesis among other causes. AFP and inhibin have no part in this evaluation. Once a work-up is complete, IM testosterone can be given to assess penile growth potential.

4. A 16-year-old boy with sickle-cell disease presents with a painful erection of 6 h duration. Initial treatment should be:

   (a) Hydration, pain control, and exchange transfusion
   (b) Winter's shunt followed by a Quackels shunt if necessary

(c) Saline irrigation and intracavernosal papaverine injection

(d) Saline irrigation and intracavernosal phenylephrine injection

(e) (a) and (d)

Answer: (e)   Low flow, or ischemic priapism, is common in sickle-cell disease with an incidence of 2–35%. Initial treatment should be multimodal, including transfusion and hydration along with irrigation and sympathomimetic injection. Shunt procedures should only be performed if this conservative therapy fails. Intracavernosal papaverine is likely to promote erection.

5. All of the following regarding varioceles are true except:

(a) The gonadotrophin response to gonadotrophin-releasing hormone (GnRH) stimulation is abnormally low in some children with varicocele

(b) Leydig cell atrophy is the predominant pathologic finding in teenagers undergoing surgery for varicocele

(c) A varicocele raises testicular temperature and repair of the varicocele normalizes testicular temperature

(d) The size of a varicocele has not been correlated with sperm count

(e) All of the above are true

Answer: (d)   Several studies have reported that men with larger varicoceles have greater impairment in semen parameters than men with a small varicocele. This finding is associated with the observation that increasing varicocele size may correlate with more ipsilateral testis volume loss.

6. A hydrocele as a complication of varicocele repair is least likely via which surgical approach?

(a) Palomo mass ligation technique

(b) Inguinal or subinguinal approach with microscopic ligation of all venous channels

(c) Laparoscopic mass ligation

(d) Intrascrotal approach

(e) None of the above

Answer: (b)   Mass ligation of the testicular artery, vein, and lymphatic channels is associated with a 10–20% risk of developing a hydrocele postoperatively. The inguinal or subinguinal approach, where the testicular artery is preserved, along with at least a single lymphatic, rarely results in a hydrocele on follow-up.

7. All of the following are true regarding the evaluation of a child with acute testicular torsion except:

(a) Absent cremasteric reflex

(b) A high-riding testis with an abnormal (transverse) lie

(c) Presence of a color Doppler signal, even in small testes, is highly accurate in ruling out torsion

(d) A history of scrotal trauma is common

(e) All of the above are true

Answer: (c)   Doppler signals in small testes of young children must be interpreted carefully. Presence of color dots does not accurately predict the presence of normal flow and a wave form within the substance of the testis must be seen.

Hiep T Nguyen

1. A 24-h-old male infant is noted to have an enlarged right hemiscrotum. It does not trans-illuminate, is not reducible, and is not tender to palpation. The most likely diagnosis is:

   (a) Direct inguinal hernia
   (b) Intravaginal testicular torsion
   (c) Extravaginal testicular torsion
   (d) Hydrocele
   (e) Yolk sac testicular tumor

   Answer: (c) This patient is likely to have extravaginal testicular torsion. Approximately 10% of all testicular torsion occurs in new-borns. In 70% of these patients, torsion occurs prenatally. Testicular torsion in newborns occurs extravaginally, where the entire sper-matic cord twists en masse. Salvage of the torsed testis is uncommon and the role of con-tralateral orchidopexy is controversial.

2. A 7-year-old girl presents with symptoms and findings consistent with a right hernia. She is scheduled for bilateral hernia repair. Which of the following procedures should be done in conjunction with her hernia repair?

   (a) Chromosomal analysis
   (b) Fluorescence in situ hybridization (FISH) test
   (c) Vaginoscopy
   (d) Diagnostic laparoscopy
   (e) No other additional tests are required

   Answer: (c) In approximately 2–3% of phenotypic girls undergoing hernia repair, a testis may be found in the sac, suggesting the

diagnosis of complete androgen insensitivity syndrome. Vaginoscopy provides a reliable method to determine the presence of a cervix, which rules out the above syndrome.

3. A 6-month-old infant underwent bilateral hernia repair without complications. In follow-up he was noted to have bilateral recurrence. His testes are otherwise normal but definite inguinal bulges are noted on physical examination. What would be the most appropriate next step?

   (a) Schedule to redo bilateral hernia repair
   (b) Observation to see if it will spontaneously resolve
   (c) Evaluation for possible etiology of recurrent hernia such as connective tissue disease
   (d) Schedule for bilateral hydrocele repair through a scrotal approach

   Answer: (c) The recurrence rate following open hernia repair is approximately 1–3%, but can be as high as 20% in premature infants. Recurrence may be due to technical problems such as failure to dissect a complete sac, tear-ing of the sac, or slipped sutures in ligating the sac. However, other pathologies such as con-nective tissue disease or abdominal ascites may account for recurrence. Technical problems are less likely to occur on both sides.

4. A 1-month-old boy presents with a right scrotal swelling that has been present since birth. The rest of genital exam is normal

without evidence of hypospadias and both testes can be palpated in the scrotum. The parents indicated that there has not been an inguinal swelling or significant variation in the size of the scrotal swelling. The most appropriate recommendation is:

(a) Schedule for bilateral hernia repair as soon as possible
(b) Reassure parents and discharge from further follow-up
(c) Suggest subsequent follow-up to see if the hydrocele resolves
(d) Perform inguinal ultrasonography to determine if a hernia is present

Answer: (c)   The symptoms and findings are most consistent with a hydrocele. Unlike hernia, hydroceles may resolve spontaneously during the first year of life. Follow-up is recommend to treat the hydrocele if it does not resolve. Ultrasonography is neither sensitive nor specific enough to diagnose the presence or absence of a hernia.

5. A 14-year-old boy presents with a 4h history of right testicular pain. It developed acutely and was associated with nausea and vomiting. The pain has been intense for most of the day and continues to be so. On physical exam, the right testis is very tender to palpation and is high-riding. The cremasteric reflex is absent on the right and present on the left. Urinalysis was negative for esterase, nitrites, and heme. The most appropriate next step is:

(a) Take the patient immediately to the operating room for scrotal exploration and possible bilateral orchidopexy
(b) Perform a testicular ultrasonography to evaluate for the presence of blood flow
(c) Treat the patient with anti-inflammatory medication and scrotal elevation

(d) Perform an abdominal and pelvic computerized tomography to evaluate for metastatic nodal disease
(e) Observe the patient to see if the pain improves with intravenous narcotics

Answer: (a)   The symptoms and findings are consistent with acute testicular torsion. The patient should be taken immediate to surgery without the need for obtaining confirmatory imaging study, in order to maximize the chance of testicular salvage.

6. A 3-week-old boy presents with a 2 day history of right groin swelling. The infant has been irritable and not feeding well during the last 2 days, though there has been no vomiting. On examination, the right testis is absent in the scrotum while the left testis is descended in the lower portion of the scrotum, and is of normal size and consistency. A firm bulge is noted in the right groin which does not reduce. Which of the following is the most likely diagnosis?

(a) Congenital absence of the right testis
(b) Torsion of the right undescended testis
(c) A cord hydrocele
(d) Right testicular appendiceal torsion

Answer: (b)   The symptoms and findings are most consistent with testicular torsion of an undescended testis. Extravaginal torsion can occur in the undescended testis. This should be suspected in a child with an absent scrotal testis and symptoms consistent with torsion.

7. A 12-year-old boy presents with several months history of intermittent left testicular pain. The pain developed acutely, usually early in the morning waking him from sleep. The pain resolved within 15–30 min. It appears to be more frequent over the last month. He denies any history of trauma, dysuria, or hematuria. He has been evaluated in the past

for these episodes, usually when the pain has resolved. Urinalysis and testicular ultrasonography were both normal. What is the most appropriate management for this patient?

(a) NSAIDs and scrotal elevation
(b) Repeat testicular ultrasound examination
(c) Schedule for bilateral orchidopexy
(d) Reassurance to parents that this likely represents benign orchalgia associated with puberty
(e) Schedule for left hernia repair

Answer: (c) The patient's history and symptoms are worrisome for intermittent testicular torsion and consequently orchidopexy would be indicated. Boys with intermittent testicular torsion typically present with a history of intermittent testicular pain which becomes more frequent and severe, culminating in an episode of acute testicular torsion. Physical exam and imaging of the testis is typically normal when the pain has resolved.

8. A 14-year-old boy presents with an asymptomatic left Grade 3 varicocele. He is a Tanner Stage IV with symmetrical testes size and normal consistency. What is the most appropriate treatment?

(a) Serial follow-up examination of testes size and, when he is older and it is appropriate, obtain a semen analysis
(b) Discharge from further follow-up care since it is a normal finding without any significant clinical sequelae
(c) Artery-sparing high ligation varicocelectomy
(d) Microscopic subinguinal varicocelectomy
(e) Percutaneous sclerosis of the varicocele

Answer: (a) Currently, the indication for surgical intervention of adolescent varicocele is for symptoms such as pain. More relative indications include marked testicular volume differential, abnormal semen parameters (when available and properly standardized), and size. In the absence of symptoms, it is quite controversial whether adolescent varicocele requires immediate treatment.

9. A 16-year-old boy has a left Grade 3 varicocele and a 50% discrepancy between the size of the left and right testes. After a thorough discussion with his parents about the potential benefits of surgical correction, they elected for him to proceed with varicocelectomy using the Palomo technique. Eight months later, the varicocele is no longer present but a left hydrocele is detected. The hydrocele was not noted at the 3 month postoperative visit. Which of the following statements is true?

(a) Since the hydrocele was not present at 3 months postvaricocelectomy, it is unlikely that the left hydrocele is related to the varicocele repair
(b) The chance of developing a hydrocele postoperatively is greater when using the microscopic subinguinal technique compared to the Palomo and Ivanissevich techniques
(c) It is not likely that the hydrocele will resolve with observation or simple scrotal puncture
(d) Recurrence following varicocele repair is usually noted several months after surgery rather than several years
(e) A higher recurrence rate of the varicocele is seen when performing mass ligation compared with artery-sparing surgery

Answer: (e) Hydroceles are infrequently detected within 6 months of varicocele repair, but more commonly at 6 months up to 3 years. The microscopic subinguinal technique has a low risk of hydrocele (0.8% versus 5–10%). Approximately 80% of patients with a hydrocele postvaricocelectomy will resolve spontaneously or following simple scrotal puncture. A lower rate of recurrence is seen with the mass ligation technique compared to the artery-sparing surgery.

10. A 12-year-old boy presents with a right Grade 2 varicocele. He has no testicular asymmetry and is asymptomatic. What would be the most appropriate management?

   (a) Observation since the patient is asymptomatic and there is no testicular discrepancy

   (b) Perform testicular ultrasonography to more accurately evaluate testicular volume
   (c) Obtain further imaging of the abdomen/pelvis and venous system
   (d) Recommend varicocele repair

Answer: (c)   Approximately 90% of the varicocele occurs on the left side and 2–10% occurs bilaterally. Isolated right-side varicocele is uncommon. Patients with right-sided varicocele require radiologic evaluation for a pelvic/abdominal mass which could compress venous return.

Cryptorchidism

74

Thomas F Kolon

1. Abnormal histology of the cryptorchid testis at 6–12 months of age includes:

   (a) Increased number of Leydig cells
   (b) Persistence of fetal gonocytes
   (c) Increased number of Sertoli cells
   (d) Early appearance of Ad spermatogonia
   (e) Early appearance of primary spermatocytes

   Answer: (b)   In the cryptorchid testis, the number of Leydic cells is decreased and they atrophy. The total number of germ cells is normal in cryptorchid testes; however, the number of spermatogonia remains low and does not increase with age, due to a lack of transformation of gonocytes (fetal stem cell pool) into Ad spermatogonia (adult stem cell pool).

2. Upon surgical exploration, what percentage of nonpalpable testes are present in the inguinal canal?

   (a) <10%
   (b) 10–25%
   (c) 25%
   (d) 50%
   (e) >50%

   Answer (e) Upon surgical exploration, 60–80% of nonpalpable testes are present in the inguinal canal or intraabdominal location. The other 20–40% of testes are absent or a nubbin.

3. Which technique is the most reliable mode of detecting an undescended testis?

   (a) Physical exam by a pediatric urologist
   (b) Physical exam by a primary care physician
   (c) Ultrasound
   (d) Doppler ultrasound
   (e) Computerized tomography (CT) scan

   Answer: (a)   Ultrasonography and CT scan both show very low reliability for detecting intraabdominal testes. Despite the higher reliability in detecting an undescended testis in a physical exam by a pediatric urologist in one study, the accuracy of a physical exam is still only 84%. Ultimately, surgical exploration is still required to rule out the presence of a testis when it is nonpalpable.

4. In the first step of testicular maturation:

   (a) Primordial germ cells enter the testicular cords and differentiate into gonocytes
   (b) Gonocytes constitute the adult stem cell pool
   (c) Müllerian inhibiting substance (MIS) stimulates fetal Leydig cell development
   (d) MIS causes regression of Wolffian duct and development of Müllerian structures
   (e) Gonocytes differentiate into primary spermatocytes

   Answer: (a)   The first step of testicular maturation is marked by the primordial germ cells entering the testicular cords and differentiating into gonocytes (fetal stem cell pool). MIS is secreted by the Sertoli cells and does cause regression of Müllerian structures and development of the Wolffian duct. Leydig cells proliferate with the surge of luteinizing hormone (LH) and follicle-stimulating hormone (FSH), and not MIS.

5. Genes that have been associated with cryptorchidism in animal gene knock-out models include all except:

   (a) Homeobox (HOX)
   (b) G-protein-coupled receptor affecting testis descent (GREAT)
   (c) Cystic fibrosis transmembrane conductance regulator (CFTR)
   (d) Calcitonin gene related peptide (CGRP)
   (e) Androgen receptor (AR)

   Answer: (c)   Homeobox (HOX) genes play a key role in the morphogenesis of segmental structures along the anterior–posterior body axis, and a knock-out in male mice is associated with bilateral cryptorchidism. GREAT gene is highly associated with the development of the gubernaculums. It is believed that calcitonin gene-related peptide (CGRP) indirectly mediates androgen-dependent inguinoscrotal descent and the androgen receptor gene (AR) is similarly involved.

6. A phenotypic boy is born with a normal-appearing penis and bilateral nonpalpable cryptorchidism. A complete evaluation should include:

   (a) Karyotype
   (b) Human chorionic gonadotrophin (hCG) stimulation test, LH, FSH
   (c) hCG stimulation test
   (d) (b) and (c)
   (e) (a) and (c)

   Answer: (d)   For a neonate <3 months of age with bilateral nonpalpable testes, the LH, FSH and testosterone levels should be checked to determine the presence of testes. In infants >3 months of age in whom LH and FSH may have returned to prepubertal levels, an hCG stimulation test will aid in diagnosis of absent testes.

7. Hormonal and laparoscopic evaluation in this same boy confirms bilateral anorchia. The testes likely atrophied at:

   (a) Conception
   (b) 4–6 weeks gestation
   (c) 6–8 weeks gestation
   (d) 8–12 weeks gestation
   (e) >12 weeks gestation

   Answer: (e)   It is generally accepted that since male differentiation of the genital tract has occurred, testicular tissue must have been present and functioning during early fetal life up to at least the 12th week of gestation. This is consistent with the association with a blind-ending spermatic cord, as the presence of the spermatic cord structure supports the testis being present during early intrauterine life.

8. When considering hCG treatment to induce testicular descent in cryptorchidism, all of the following are true except:

   (a) Distal inguinal testes in older boys are more likely to respond
   (b) Repeated courses offer little advantage
   (c) Side-effects of hCG include increased scrotal rugae and pubic hair
   (d) A total dose up to 25 000 IU can safely be given to avoid epiphyseal growth plate closure
   (e) Long-term success rates in controlled studies appear to be about 20%

   Answer: (d)   A total hCG dose should be kept <15 000 IU, since it may induce epiphyseal plate fusion and retard future somatic growth.

9. Development of testicular histology and endocrine function begins during:

   (a) The 4th gestational week
   (b) Gestational weeks 5–6

(c) The 7th gestational week

(d) Abdominal testicular descent

(e) Inguinoscrotal testicular descent

Answer: (c)   Development of testicular histology and endocrine function begins during the 7th gestational week and continues into adulthood. It is characterized by four steps in maturation prior to the final maturational changes at puberty.

10. Obstetric risk factors for cryptorchidism include:

(a) Young maternal age

(b) Low parity

(c) Low birth weight

(d) (b) and (c)

(e) (a), (b) and (c)

Answer: (d)   Young maternal age is not correlated with the risk of cryptorchidism, while low parity and low birth weight of the infant increases the risk for cryptorchidism.

Surgical management of the undescended testis

75

Israel Franco

1. The percentage of testicles which will descend spontaneously after a boy is 6 months of age is:

   (a) <10%
   (b) 10–20%
   (c) 20–30%
   (d) 30–40%
   (e) 40–50%

   Answer: (a) According to a study by Wenzler et al only 6.9% of all testes will descend spontaneously after a boy is 6 months of age.[1]

2. In utero torsion is more likely to occur on:

   (a) Right side
   (b) Left side
   (c) Both sides
   (d) Occurs infrequently
   (e) Occurs only in premies

   Answer: (b) In utero torsion tends to occur more often on the left side with reported incidences of 70–90%. Bilateral in utero torsion is extremely rare occurring in an estimated 1:20 000 births.

3. The diagnosis of testicular in utero torsion is best made in the operative field by the presence of:

   (a) Hemosiderin
   (b) Cartilage
   (c) Fibrosis
   (d) Greenish-brown discoloration of the testis
   (e) Absence of testicular tissue

   Answer: (d) The first three answers are all microscopic diagnosis which are found in in utero torsion, but in the surgical field the only way to know there is hemorrhage present when the testes infarct is to see a greenish-brown discoloration of the tissue. Absence of testicular tissue can be misleading, since there may be a looping vas with an epididymal structure while there remains an intraabdominal testis.

4. The best place to approach the hernia sac during an open inguinal orchidopexy is:

   (a) Distal to the external inguinal ring
   (b) At the external inguinal ring
   (c) Proximal to the external inguinal ring
   (d) At the internal inguinal ring
   (e) There is no need to take the hernia sac

   Answer: (d) The best place to take the hernia sac is at the internal inguinal ring. Here the sac is the narrowest, and generally leads to the least amount of dissection on and around the gonadal vessels and vas. The sac is easily delineated by its white color on the medial side when it is adjacent to the preperitoneal fat that is present along the cord.

5. The best procedure to help identify a nonpalpable testis is:

   (a) Ultrasound of the scrotum
   (b) Ultrasound of the abdomen

(c) Computerized tomography (CT) scan of the abdomen and pelvis

(d) Magnetic resonance imaging (MRI) of the abdomen and pelvis

(e) Surgical exploration

Answer: (e) The standard at this time is surgical exploration, whether it is laparoscopy or open surgery is the preference of the surgeon. The results for radiologic procedures are poor and in the case of gadolinium-enhanced MRI the data pool is too small to make a definitive affirmation of its value.

6. During an orchidopexy the surgeon finds that there is not enough length after transecting the gubernaculum and dissecting the cord from the floor of the canal. What additional maneuvers will give the surgeon additional length and allow placement of the testis in the scrotum?

(a) Dissect the lateral spermatic fascia off the cord

(b) Utilize a Jones incision and gain access to the retroperitoneum and dissect the gonadal vessels up the posterior abdominal wall

(c) Leave the hernia sac intact and consider doing a Fowler Stephens orchidopexy in one stage

(d) Strip the cord of the hernia sac and do Fowler Stephens orchidopexy

(e) (a), (b) and (c)

Answer: (e) Any of the answers (a), (b) or (c) are correct depending on the situation. Stripping the cord of the hernia sac and interrupting the blood supply between the vas and the collaterals to the epididymis will invariably lead to failure in cases when a Fowler Stephens orchidopexy is performed. These collaterals are essential to the preservation of blood flow to the testis when the gonadal vessels are transected.

7. The most common reason for a failed orchidopexy is:

(a) Inadequate dissection of the cord

(b) Leaving a hernia sac behind

(c) Lateral placement of the testis outside the scrotum

(d) All of the above

(e) None of the above

Answer: (c) The most common reason for a failed orchidopexy is the placement of the testis lateral to the scrotum. The surgeon will typically follow the path of the testis, which was ectopically placed, and try to make the subdartos pouch via this lateral approach, and thereby be destined to have the testis migrate out of the scrotum.

8. Testicular autotransplantation is carried out by anastomosing the gonadal vessels to the:

(a) Inferior epigastric vessels

(b) Superficial circumflex iliac vessels

(c) Superficial pudendal vessels

(d) Femoral vessels

(e) Any of the above

Answer: (a) The inferior epigastric vessels are mobilized for 8–9 cm beneath the rectus muscle towards the umbilicus. The distal end is ligated and the proximal end is clipped. The proximal vessels are then irrigated with heparinized saline and the anastomosis is completed to the gonadal vessels.

9. In a one-stage Fowler Stephens orchidopexy the most important step in the operation is:

(a) High ligation of the gonadal vessels

(b) Distal ligation of the gonadal vessels as per Koff

(c) Complete mobilization of the cord and stripping of the vas and vessels distally near the epididymis to get as much length as possible

(d) Avoid manipulation of the epididymis and vas, maintaining the small vessels between the two

(e) All of the above

Answer: (d) Maintaining the blood supply that exists in the adventitial tissue between the vas and the epididymis is essential to a successful Fowler Stephens orchidopexy. It does not appear to make a difference if the vessels are ligated distally or proximally as long as the collateral blood supply is maintained.

10. A common complication during laparoscopic orchidopexy during the delivery of the testis out of the abdomen is:

(a) Injury to the femoral veins

(b) Injury to the bladder

(c) Avulsion of the medial umbilical ligament

(d) Ureteral obstruction

(e) Hernia formation at the site

Answer: (a) Injury to the bladder is by far the most common injury other than initial trocar injuries. This is most likely to occur if the surgeon fails to leave the bladder decompressed during the whole case. Injury to the femoral vessels is more common if an approach is taken that takes you lateral to the median umbilical ligament. Ureteral obstruction has occurred but it is due to inadequate dissection of the peritoneum from the ureter at or near the root of the small bowel mesentery. Only one report of a hernia has been described to date but this was at the native internal ring.

11. Injury to the bladder can be avoided by:

(a) Making sure that a catheter is left in the bladder at all times during the case

(b) Making sure that the instrument making the path is driven from the ipsilateral side in a medial direction

(c) Minimize the dissection at the pubic bone

(d) Do not strip the peritoneum off the gonadal vessels

(e) Sew the hiatus closed after the testis has been delivered outside the abdomen

Answer: (a) The bladder should be left decompressed the whole time to minimize the risk of bladder injury and to facilitate dissection of the vas off the bladder wall. Not removing the peritoneum off the gonadal vessels will lead to insufficient length in many cases and possible ascent of the testis after the orchidopexy.

Reference

1. Wenzler D et al. What is the rate of spontaneous testicular descent in infants with cryptorchidism? J Urol 2004; 171: 849–51.

Testicular tumors

76

Jonathan H Ross

1. When compared to testicular tumors occurring in adults, testicular tumors in children are:

   (a) More likely to be benign
   (b) More likely to have a mixed pathology
   (c) Less likely to present as a testicular mass
   (d) More likely to have an elevated serum beta-human chorionic gonadotrophin (hCG) level
   (e) When malignant, more likely to require retroperitoneal lymph node dissection (RPLND) and/or chemotherapy following orchiectomy

   Answer: (a)   Children have a higher incidence of benign tumors (most often teratoma) and rarely have mixed germ cell tumors. When malignant, the large majority are managed with observation without chemotherapy and RPLND is almost never employed. The overwhelming number of malignant tumors in children are yolk sac tumors which produce alphafetoprotein (AFP), but not beta-hCG. Most tumors present as a testicular mass.

2. The most important role for ultrasound in evaluating children with a scrotal mass is:

   (a) Distinguishing benign from malignant tumors
   (b) Distinguishing testicular from extratesticular lesions
   (c) Determining whether testis-sparing surgery is possible
   (d) Determining whether the lesion is hypervascular or hypovascular
   (e) Providing information for local staging of a tumor

   Answer: (b)   Ultrasound is very accurate in distinguishing testicular from extratesticular lesions. While ultrasound can detect cystic changes which occur more commonly in benign lesions, it cannot reliably make the distinction between benign and malignant tumors. It can also be misleading with regard to the feasibility of testis-sparing surgery as even large lesions may be enucleated leaving a reasonable amount of normal parenchyma. Ultrasound is not routinely used for staging or determining the vascularity of a lesion.

3. The best management for a 2-month-old boy with a testicular tumor and a serum AFP level of 300 ng/ml is:

   (a) Close observation with serial ultrasounds, physical exams and AFP levels
   (b) Inguinal orchiectomy with RPLND
   (c) Inguinal orchiectomy without RPLND
   (d) Tumor excision with further management based on frozen section analysis
   (e) Trans-scrotal needle biopsy

   Answer: (d)   An AFP of 300 ng/ml is normal in a 2-month-old boy and so the tumor is most likely benign. Therefore, an inguinal exploration with excisional biopsy and frozen section analysis is appropriate. If a benign histology is confirmed, then nothing further need be done. If the tumor is malignant, the orchiectomy can be completed.

4. A 1-year-old boy undergoes orchiectomy for a yolk sac tumor. His computerized tomography (CT) scan of the chest and abdomen is normal and his serum AFP which was initially 5200 ng/ml decreases to 120 ng/ml at 4 weeks postoperatively. The best management is:

(a) Close observation with frequent radiographic and biochemical follow-up
(b) Four courses of platinum-based chemotherapy
(c) Modified ipsilateral RPLND with further therapy based on the pathological results
(d) Bilateral RPLND with further therapy based on the pathological results
(e) No oncologic follow-up or treatment

Answer: (a) While the AFP is still slightly elevated, it is decreasing as expected based on a half-life of 5 days. Therefore, the patient has stage 1 disease which is best managed with close observation followed by chemotherapy if there is a recurrence.

5. A 1-year-old boy undergoes orchiectomy for a yolk sac tumor. His CT scan of the chest is normal. His CT scan of the abdomen reveals one enlarged ipsilateral retroperitoneal lymph node measuring 5 cm. His AFP which was initially 5600 ng/ml decreases to 3000 ng/ml at 4 weeks postoperatively. The best management is:

(a) Close observation with frequent radiographic and biochemical follow-up
(b) Four courses of platinum-based chemotherapy
(c) Modified ipsilateral RPLND with further therapy based on the pathological results
(d) Bilateral retroperitoneal lymph node biopsy with further therapy based on the pathological results
(e) Four courses of chemotherapy including actinomycin and vincristine

Answer: (b) This patient has metastatic disease based on his CT scan and failure of his AFP to drop at a rate commensurate with a half-life of 5 days. The standard therapy is three to four courses of platinum-based chemotherapy. An RPLND would be indicated only if he had a persistent mass despite normal markers following chemotherapy – a rare occurrence.

6. A 3-year-old boy undergoes an orchiectomy for a testicular mass. The final pathology reveals mature teratoma. The next step in management is:

(a) A CT scan of the chest, abdomen, and pelvis
(b) Four courses of platinum-based chemotherapy
(c) Staging RPLND
(d) (a) and (c)
(e) No further evaluation or therapy

Answer: (e) Mature teratomas are universally benign in prepubertal patients.

7. A 7-year-old boy presents with precocious puberty and a testicular mass. Which of the following is true regarding the best management of this patient:

(a) If his serum 17-hydroxyprogesterone level is high then he should be treated with corticosteroids and tumor excision
(b) If his serum 17-hydroxyprogesterone level is high then he should be treated with an orchiectomy and no corticosteroids
(c) If his serum 17-hydroxyprogesterone level is high then he should be treated initially with corticosteroids and no tumor excision
(d) He will likely require chemotherapy
(e) He will likely require bilateral orchiectomy with androgen replacement therapy at puberty

Answer: (c) The differential diagnosis is congenital adrenal hyperplasia (CAH) versus a Leydig cell tumor. If the 17-hydroxyprogesterone level is high then he likely has CAH and should be treated with corticosteroids. The testicular nodules usually regress in this setting, though excisional biopsy is occasionally required if they persist. If the patient has a Leydig cell tumor it may be treated with testis-sparing excision, particularly if bilateral.

8. An 8-year-old boy with abnormal mucocutaneous pigmentation and hamartomatous intestinal polyposis undergoes an orchiectomy for a testicular tumor. The testis tumor histopathology typical of patients with these clinical characteristics is:

   (a) Yolk sac tumor
   (b) Teratoma
   (c) Large cell calcifying Sertoli cell tumor
   (d) Leydig cell tumor
   (e) Juvenile granulose cell tumor

   Answer: (c)   The patient has the stigmata of Peutz-Jeghers syndrome which is associated with large cell calcifying Sertoli cell tumors of the testis (as is Carney's syndrome).

9. A newborn boy with an abnormal Y chromosome is found to have a testicular tumor. This tumor is most likely:

   (a) Hormonally active and benign
   (b) Hormonally active and malignant
   (c) Hormonally inactive and benign
   (d) Hormonally inactive and multifocal
   (e) Malignant and multifocal

   Answer: (c)   The most common newborn testicular tumors are juvenile granulosa cell tumors and yolk sac tumors. Patients with juvenile granulosa cell tumors often have abnormalities of the Y chromosome and mosaicism.

10. Which of the following patients should undergo prophylactic gonadectomy due to the risk of malignant degeneration:

    (a) A 3-year-old girl with Turner's syndrome
    (b) A 46XX child with pure gonadal dysgenesis
    (c) A 46XY child with pure gonadal dysgenesis
    (d) (b) and (c)
    (e) None of the above

    Answer: (c)   Patients with dysgenetic gonads and a Y chromosome in their karyotype are at high risk for gonadoblastomas (which can degenerate into malignant germ cell tumors). Patients with Turner's syndrome (who have 45XO karyotypes) and 46XX pure gonadal dysgenesis are not at significant risk.

Gordon A McLorie

(Based on chapter written by Gordon A McLorie and Darius J Bagli)

1. The best prognostic feature for children presenting with neuroblastoma is:

   (a) n-myc amplifications
   (b) Less than 1 year at presentation
   (c) Presence of Homer-Wright pseudo-rosettes in histology
   (d) Alterations in chromosome 3 or 11

   Answer: (b)   Patients diagnosed at 1 year of age appear to show consistently better survival outcomes than older children, even in the presence of advanced disease at presentation. Abnormal rearrangements of chromosomes 1 and 17, and amplification of n-myc proto-oncogene, have been implicated in poor survival. Homer-Wright pseudorossettes are histologically diagnostic of neuroblastoma, characterized by eosinophilic neutrophils surrounded by neuroblasts (occur in 50% of cases).

2. Infants with sacrococcygeal tumors presenting in infancy:

   (a) Are best treated by surgical excision in infancy
   (b) Are best treated by multimodality treatment regimens
   (c) Often have hormonal disturbances
   (d) Should be investigated for distant meta-stases

   Answer: (a)   Sacrococcygeal teratomas, the most common neoplasm in the newborn, are now commonly diagnosed antenatally, with the majority of those diagnosed prior to 1 year of age being benign. Complete en bloc removal of the tumor with the involved portion of the coccyx is the treatment of choice.

3. With pheochromocytoma in children, which of the following statements are true?

   (a) Ratio of norepinephrine to epinephrine is helpful in distinguishing origin
   (b) Metaiodobenzylguanidine (MIBG) scan is helpful in distinguishing origin
   (c) Alpha-adrenergic receptor blockade is important in surgical therapy
   (d) All of the above

   Answer: (d)   Pheochromocytomas, particularly of adrenal origin, catalyze the conversion of norepinephrine to epinephrine, so the ratio distinguishes whether tumors are of adrenal or extraadrenal origin. MIBG is the most specific diagnostic imaging modality to diagnose pheochromocytoma. Alpha-adrenergic blockade often combined with cardiac beta blockade to control reflex tachycardia remains a mainstay of preoperative preparation.

Tissue engineering applications in pediatric urology

78

Anthony Atala

1. Challenges for the engineering of normal pediatric urologic tissues include:

   (a) An adequate cell source
   (b) Adequate biomaterials
   (c) Adequate vascularization
   (d) All of the above
   (e) None of the above

   Answer: (d)   This question underlies some of the major challenges in the field of tissue engineering. Adequate cell sources, biomaterials, and vascularization are all required for the successful engineering of tissues.

2. The use of biomaterials:

   (a) Facilitates the localization and delivery of cells
   (b) Facilitates the localization and delivery of bioactive factors
   (c) Defines a three-dimensional space for the formation of new tissues
   (d) Guides the development of new tissues with appropriate function
   (e) All of the above

   Answer: (e)   A biomaterial is essential for most applications in the field of tissue engineering. Biomaterials can be used for cell attachment, to define the three-dimensional space of the new tissue or to guide the development of the new tissues. Biomaterials can be either implanted or injected.

3. Inert biomaterials without cells can regenerate normal tissue when addressing:

   (a) Defects up to 0.5 cm in diameter
   (b) Defects up to 1.0 cm in diameter
   (c) Defects up to 2.0 cm in diameter
   (d) Defects up to 5.0 cm in diameter
   (e) Defects of all sizes

   Answer: (b)   The current limit of normal tissue regeneration using biomaterials alone is 1 cm. Defects >1 cm usually require the use of biomaterials and cells for normal tissue development without fibrosis or scar formation.

4. When inert biomaterials are used without cells it could lead to:

   (a) Abnormal collagen deposition
   (b) Abnormal fibroblast deposition
   (c) Scar formation
   (d) Graft contracture
   (e) All of the above

   Answer: (e)   Several pathologic events may result when biomaterials are used without cells to cover defects >1 cm in diameter. These findings may include extensive collagen and fibroblast deposition, scar formation, and eventual graft contracture.

5. Which approach has been used for the vascularization of engineered tissue?

   (a) Incorporation of angiogenic factors in the bioengineered tissue

(b) Seeding extracellular matrix (ECM) with various cell types in the bioengineered tissue

(c) Prevascularization of the matrix prior to cell seeding

(d) All of the above

(e) None of the above

Answer: (d) One of the restrictions of the engineering of tissues is that cells cannot be implanted in volumes exceeding $3\,mm^3$ because of the limitations of nutrition and gas exchange. To achieve the goals of engineering large complex tissues and possibly internal organs, vascularization of the regenerating tissue is essential. All of the approaches listed have been used for vascularization of bioengineered tissue.

6. The preferred cell source for tissue engineering currently involves:

(a) Human embryonic stem cells

(b) Heterologous adult cells

(c) Autologous native cells

(d) Bone marrow stem cells

(e) All of the above

Answer: (c) There are many sources of cells which can be used for tissue engineering. However, the preferred source still remains autologous native cells. Native cells do not elicit an immune rejection response and they need minimal manipulation for terminal differentiation.

7. Genetically normal progenitor cells, which are the reservoirs for new cell formation, are programmed to give rise to:

(a) Other progenitor cells, regardless of whether the niche resides in either normal or diseased tissues

(b) Normal cells, regardless of whether the niche resides in either normal or diseased tissues

(c) Other progenitor cells, but only if the niche resides in normal tissue

(d) Normal cells, but only if the niche resides in normal tissue

(e) None of the above

Answer: (b) Most tissue types in the body have been shown to have progenitor cell niches. The progenitor cell niche gives rise to normal cells which are expanded during normal regeneration in response to injury or disease. Although epigenetic changes may occur, the cells are genetically normal and usually retain their function.

8. Therapeutic cloning:

(a) Can be used to generate embryonic stem cell lines which will not be rejected

(b) Has been banned in most countries

(c) Was used to clone the first mammal, a sheep named Dolly

(d) Is a technique used to generate genetically unmatched material different from its source

(e) All of the above

Answer: (a) Two types of nuclear cloning – reproductive cloning and therapeutic cloning – have been described. Banned in most countries for human applications, reproductive cloning is used to generate an embryo that has the identical genetic material to its cell source. This embryo can then be implanted into the uterus of a female to give rise to an infant that is a clone of the donor. On the other hand, therapeutic cloning is used to generate early stage embryos that are explanted in culture to produce embryonic stem cell lines that are genetically identical to the source.

Index

T - #0606 - 071024 - C0 - 254/190/13 - PB - 9780367386894 - Gloss Lamination